On the Dark Side of the Moon:

A journey toward recovery

On the Dark Side of the Moon:
A journey toward recovery

Mike Medberry

Caxton Press
Caldwell, Idaho
2012

ISBN 978-087004-513-4

Library of Congress Cataloging-in-Publication Data

Medberry, Mike.
  On the dark side of the moon : a journey toward recovery / Mike Medberry.
    pages ; cm
  ISBN 978-0-87004-513-4
  1. Medberry, Mike--Health. 2. Cerebrovascular disease--Patients--
Rehabilitation. 3. Cerebrovascular disease--Patients--Idaho--
Biography. 4. Craters of the Moon National Monument (Idaho)
I. Title.

  RC388.5.M437 2012
  616.810092--dc23
  [B]

                2012037606

Lithographed and bound in the United States of America
Caxton Press
Caldwell, Idaho

                182719

I want to tell what the forests
were like
I will have to speak
in a forgotten language

- W.S. Merwin, "Witness"

Table of Contents

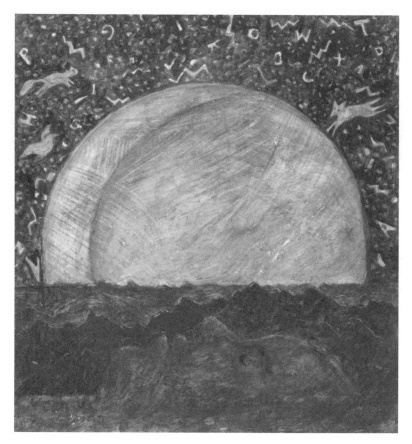

Original artwork by
Kim Howard.

Dedication

To Marj Medberry, Merritt Frey, Sue Randle, Katie Alvord, and my canine companion Camas, for all of their love and kindess.

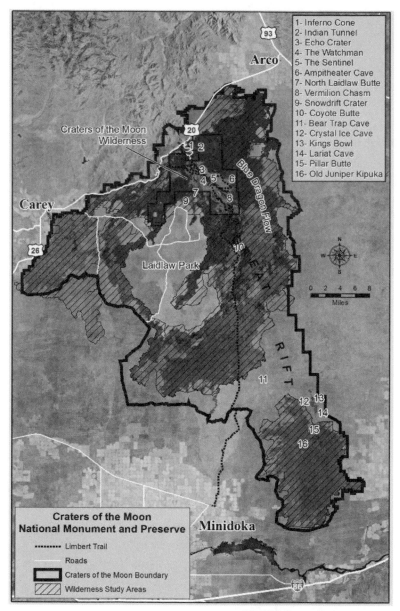

1- Inferno Cone
2- Indian Tunnel
3- Echo Crater
4- The Watchman
5- The Sentinel
6- Ampitheater Cave
7- North Laidlaw Butte
8- Vermilion Chasm
9- Snowdrift Crater
10- Coyote Butte
11- Bear Trap Cave
12- Crystal Ice Cave
13- Kings Bowl
14- Lariat Cave
15- Pillar Butte
16- Old Juniper Kipuka

Arco

Craters of the Moon
Wilderness

Carey

Blue Dragon Flow

Laidlaw Park

RIFT

**Craters of the Moon
National Monument and Preserve**

Minidoka

········· Limbert Trail

——— Roads

▭ Craters of the Moon Boundary

▨ Wilderness Study Areas

0 2 4 6 8
Miles

map courtesy of Spatial Dynamics Inc.

Chapter One

Craters of the Moon

Taking a stroll in Craters of the Moon National Monument and Preserve in southeast Idaho, near Carey, is to walk on the dark side of the moon. It is distant, lonely, alien, and fabulous beyond belief. The contrast of black lava against the cobalt-blue sky is stunning, but it is a rugged and deserted scene, a landscape of shattered saucers and teacups of broken lava that clatter with every step. Fifty-four miles north to south and 25 miles east to west, this vast national monument and preserve harbors no flowing rivers or creeks. The solidified lava reaches 140 degrees or more in the summer and subzero temperatures in winter. This was the place that Washington Irving had described in *The Adventures of Captain Bonneville*, "where nothing meets the eye but a desolate and awful waste; where no grass grows nor water runs, and where nothing is to be seen but lava."

Craters of the Moon is a hell of a place to be stranded and facing death. In the long run, however, I saw more than a harrowing world. I found more than a desolation of black rock and awful waste; I felt weightless for awhile there on the moon, paralyzed, and speechless as Craters of the Moon nursed me back to life on solid ground. Great beauty abounds in this rocky world, and it became a place to think, to reflect on losses,

1

and to define what it means to recover, both the land and myself.

I visited this area in early April 2000 with three friends— Miguel Fredes, Doug Schnitzspahn, and Katie Fite. I worked for the non-profit organization, American Lands as their public lands director and advocated protection of public lands in Idaho and across the West. I was the former public lands director of the Idaho Conservation League for seven years. Katie, who worked for the Committee for Idaho's High Deserts, and I had met with Molly McUsic, counselor to Interior Secretary Bruce Babbitt, in late 1999 in Washington, D.C. Katie and I aimed to gain protection for the Owyhee Canyonlands as a half-million acre wilderness with several scenic rivers in southwest Idaho. However, Ms. McUsic caught us off-guard by asking what we thought about enlarging the Craters of the Moon area as a national monument. Both Katie and I knew the region but we downplayed the importance of Craters of the Moon, as we didn't perceive it as being in danger of development. I thought that the beauty was less than what we advocated in the Canyonlands area, but I promised to send Ms. McUsic as much information as I had on Craters. Now President Clinton was considering adding 750,000 acres to the already designated 54,000 acre national monument, and Sec. Babbitt would soon arrive with geologists and political allies to assess the landscape. I had hiked there three times over the previous ten years and knew what I wanted to show Babbitt. And I knew that Babbitt's proposal would raise considerable opposition that would require support from conservationists.

The four of us intended to gather information about issues sure to come up in public hearings on the expansion proposal, including the effects of livestock grazing, hunting, water use, and off-road vehicle use on lava formations. Granted, you couldn't do much damage to a field of parched lava, but we would check the current condition of archeological sites, caves, plants like the miniature monkey flower and dwarf buckwheat, and animals like mule deer, badger, red fox, sage grouse, pika, and pronghorn antelope. As professional conservationists, we wanted to say, "We know that land by foot, not by hearsay or speculation, and here's what we think of the proposal...."

I especially wanted to revisit Laidlaw Park, a kipuka, or an island of soil and grass surrounded by miles of lava that had issued from the Great Rift lava flow. The Great Rift volcanic zone is a wide line of open cracks in the earth, eruptive fissures, shield volcanoes, and cinder cones that extends more than 50 miles from the Pioneer Mountains near Sun Valley, Idaho to the Wapi Lava Field by Pocatello. The Great Rift and Laidlaw Park were outside of the original monument and the Idaho Conservation League had proposed both as additions to the monument in 1990. At 50,000 acres, the Laidlaw Park kipuka is the largest in the United States, supporting many unusual plants and animals. Parched, fertile, and remote, it is open only to limited livestock grazing and is less damaged than most of America's public lands.

We drove three and a half hours from Boise and turned onto a remote road between the small towns of Carey and Arco. We arrived at Craters at night and stayed in a scenic, but closed, campground at the edge of the national monument beside the National Park's visitor's center. I had run a half-marathon earlier that day, and was proud of finishing 88th out of 2,200 runners. But I felt thirsty as we drove away. I should have been tired and ready to turn in, but instead Doug and I stayed up late quoting poetry at each other—Dickinson, Dylan Thomas, Yeats. He and I had both been MFA students at the

University of Washington and were pretentious writers as well as conservationists.

In the morning, I decided to pick up where we left off, with a favorite, Dickinson's poem, "The Brain is wider than the Sky. Doug, remember that one?" Doug rolled up his sleeping bag. "...They will chan, diff just like syllable from, uh ..."

Doug looked oddly at me. "The brain is just the weight of God,/ For, lift them, pound for pound,/ And they will differ, if they do, /As syllable from sound." He recited the last stanza perfectly. "Man, you'd better get some coffee," he said, laughing.

On our drive through Laidlaw Park, we stopped at a junction in the road to look at what appeared to be a small volcano, Big Blowout Butte. Just then, I saw the silhouette of a bird flying on swift wing, calling—"keek, keek, keek, keek!" I watched it, mesmerized by its shallow wingbeats, as it disappeared beyond the butte, as quickly seen as gone. "Was that a peregrine or a prairie falcon?" I asked Doug, but he hadn't seen the bird. As we drove on, I marked the spot where it had headed, intending to look for it on the way out.

We parked at the far end of the road and walked for an hour over a lava flow where sagebrush grew like whiskers on a craggy face. As a boy, I'd lived for a time in Hawaii and was familiar with the various types of lava, including a'a (ah ah) and pahoehoe (pah-hoey-hoey)—Hawaiian names that convey a sense of the lava's presence. Pahoehoe is smooth and homogenous, like melted chocolate frozen in the act of flowing. A'a, with its jumbled sharp rocks, is as choppy as a hurricane sea. Many years later, when I first saw the lava fields at Craters of the Moon, they held the same lure for me as lava in Hawaii. I learned that the buttes and cindercones were different from Hawaiian volcanoes, but the oozing lava flows were much the same.

Craters of the Moon

When the path became less rugged, so I could afford to look up instead of at my feet, I saw an endless reach of pure black rock and gray stretches of rubble. In April, Craters of the Moon has a Jekyll and Hyde personality—sleety squalls storming across the land or wind bringing an icy fog, alternating with brief sunny spells. As we hiked, we experienced the full force of this metereorological schizophrenia. Hyde was in control.

We walked through an oceanic expanse of blowing grasses crashing on the rocks in the spray of wind. Katie found an archeological site that had been vandalized, so we photographed it and continued on in the misting rain across an isthmus of lava. We were on our way to the summit of Bowl Crater, which offered a sweeping vista of the potential monument. The trek was a fascinating path through a mixture of smooth, raven-black rock and tumultuous waves of grayer stone, and through all of this we had to watch every uneven and slippery step. As we stopped and gazed at the view, my head throbbed. *Where had this killer headache come from?* I asked Katie for an aspirin—no, make it two—then walked away to look out over the endless lava. The pain was excruciating and the aspirin was doing nothing to abate it.

I rejoined my friends and we headed back toward our parking spot enveloped in a gauzy, blowing fog. I looked forward to a Moosehead beer, chips with red-hot salsa, and warming my hands by the car's heater. Katie, Doug, and Miguel plodded on with their heads buried in their raincoat hoods as we crossed the stormy sea of black rock. There were no trails, but we had agreed to meet back at our cars if we lost sight of each other.

I was hop-scotching through the lava and stumbled on nothing. I suddenly had an odd feeling of weightlessness, as if floating above the ground in the fog. Then a sharp pain suddenly fell on my head like the blow of an axe. I must have passed out, because when I came to, in an indefinite time, my legs were useless, my thoughts incoherent. I had smacked my head hard on the lava, but the pain wasn't coming from the outside. It was somewhere inside, somewhere I couldn't touch. I tried to yell, "Hey, guys, wait up!" but I couldn't yell. My yells were imaginary and blocked.

What had sent me sprawling onto the lava? How had I fallen? Was it a heart attack, a gunshot, or just a hard smack on my head from falling? I couldn't catch my breath. I was a 44-year-old long-distance runner, yet I lay immobilized on the lava like a broken oyster. I drifted in and out of consciousness, in and out of pain, unable to do a damn thing.

My friends would get back to the cars and wonder about me. They'd be annoyed at having to wait. After an hour or two, maybe they'd worry and look for me, but with no trails, where would they look? Already it was late afternoon. Carey, the cowtown we'd driven through on our way to Laidlaw Park, was an hour and a half away. Even if they found me, what then? I was in trouble beyond what I could fathom. I couldn't talk, I couldn't yell, I couldn't walk or even crawl. I was reduced to gurgling like a baby and was confused beyond belief.

Inert on the lava, I tried to take inventory. I looked at the world with one good eye. Why was everything so bleary through the other? My right eye was wet and hurt like hell. It felt huge, like the monstrous eye of a Cyclops. I must have smashed it on the lava. How long had I lain there? Minutes, seconds, hours? I had no idea. My right leg wouldn't work, and my right arm was as limp as a shot rabbit. But my left leg and arm had life in them. Surely I could move and stand and walk. I managed to push up on my left arm but immediately fell. My face felt like it had been hatcheted in two. I wiped blood from my one good hand on my jeans and my bright yellow rain jacket.

I'll get out of this, I told myself. I'd gotten out of some bad scrapes before. But now something was going wrong with my brain; it was spinning as if caught in a tornado. My mind moved randomly to the past. I remembered that when I was twelve my father had a stroke. When I went to see him in the hospital, he wore a pirate's eye-patch and a white turban to hide the cut the doctors had opened in his head. He pointed, shook his finger, and grunted as he looked out the window of Tripler Army Medical Center in Honolulu, Hawaii. My father, a lawyer and Air Force colonel, had been rendered speechless. Back then, I was baffled by my feeling of helplessness due to his inability to communicate with me. But I understood that he wanted the hell out of the hospital. He died six months later.

Now I knew a piece of his death firsthand. And I wanted out of this goddamn black rock desert. I tried to sit up again but slid down the slanted piece of broken pahoehoe lava on which I was lying. I caught a branch and held on with all my strength. I feared that if I let go I would slide down into heavy brush and be completely lost from sight.

Make me whole again, I prayed to a silent God. I clung to the branch because I could feel that one thing clearly. It represented life. The fragrance of sagebrush engulfed me, sweet and bitter, the smell of rich soil, the smell of coming rain in the desert.

I passed out again and woke to see the sun shining brightly and the clouds sending out spokes of light. I passed out and woke yet again. Clouds darkened half the sky, threatening more rain as the sun began to set. My heartbeats counted out the day. I felt a pain in my chest and called out to the earth, but what use was that? The earth I'd worked 20 years to protect was silent.

A minute-long squall chilled me to the bone, and the water that collected in little depressions of the a'a evaporated in minutes, so I couldn't get a drink. Life was elemental on the lava. A spider walked by my one good eye. I tried to move, but it kept on coming until I screamed inarticulately and blew it away. How could I survive if I could barely divert a spider?

My thoughts shifted jaggedly between awareness of my body and what I needed to do. That struck me as funny: "what I need to do." I wasn't going anywhere at all, and the sun was going down. My hopes for saving this piece of land might be lost if I couldn't get the hell up and out of here. Save the land? You kidding? How was I going to do that if I couldn't save myself? The setting sun bathed me in brilliant colors: orange, scarlet, and clear, dripping yellow. I hung on to the branch. It was something of this world on which I could focus as my consciousness slipped. I felt pressure on my chest and looked up at a dark animal who stood with his heavy paws on me, pinning me to the ground. I closed my eyes and tried to make this horrible mirage disappear, but my mind whispered that it had come to me for a reason.

I became pure observer, watching the land with my one eye. I breathed heavily and deeply in the chill air and accepted that this day would be my last. I felt myself a part of this fantastic landscape, no more than the lava and no less. I gave myself to it, to its aching brightness and growing shadows, to its burning heat and its cold sleety winds. In a moment of pure calm, an unparalleled peace and balance, I felt my life in exquisite detail. Was this what it was like to die? Well, if so, dying wouldn't be so bad. Death beckoned like a smooth slide into warm water.

Yes, I was going to die soon. There was nothing I could do about it.

***

I stood at the base of the papaya tree looking up at three of the plump yellow fruits clustered under big hand-shaped leaves. My father loomed behind me, maneuvering a 12-foot pole with a snipper at the top. I loathed papaya: the slug-slime texture of the meat, the babypoo color, the mouse-turd seeds, the musty smell that made me gag.

"Son, you ready to catch?" My father positioned the snipper against the stem of the biggest papaya. "Fly ball comin' atcha."

At age 12 and an only child, I lived for baseball. I knew the difference between a flyball and a papaya. "Just cut it, Dad."

"Ready? Last time you weren't ready and you made a big mess."

"It's too ripe, Dad. Just like last time." Last week only half of one fruit had even been salvageable. He was right: big mess, most of it on me.

"Perfect papayas up there, son. You might just like 'em: a little salt, some lime, mmm—mmm—mmm!"

"Dad, please just cut the thing. My neck's getting sore."

"Ok, ok. Well, I'm glad you don't like these beautiful golden papayas then." He gave me a sideways glance and smirked. He had a big face, slightly inset eyes with dark shadows, and wispy hair. "You'll look back someday and regret that you didn't eat fresh papaya in Oahu when you had the chance. Listen to your old man."

"You're not that old, Dad. Just cut it, ok? Let's get this over with."

"Ok, here she comes." My father pulled the rope that controlled the snipper, and the papaya plummeted. I jumped back

9

out of the way as it splattered on the grass like a balloon full of yellow mush.

"Oh, goddammit, Mike." My father looked with disgust at the ruined papaya, then with disappointment at me. "What happened, son?" He put his hands on his hips, knuckles in. I thought he looked funny trying to act angry in his flowery aloha shirt and baggy swim trunks with that papaya all smashed on the ground and yellow splotches of it on his legs.

"I learned my lesson last week, Dad." I could hardly keep a straight face. "It's nothing like a fly ball. You try it."

Cutting papayas with me in our yard was my father's idea of relaxation and bonding—"teamwork," he called it. It was the summer of 1968, and he was stationed at Hickam Air Force Base in Honolulu, where we'd moved after his stints in Ohio, California, and Washington, D.C. The United States was at war in Vietnam, and as an air force attorney and colonel, he was working on contracts for private companies to supply military bases in Southeast Asia.

Despite his goofball moments, my dad was invincible in my eyes. His full name was John Raymond Medberry, but everyone called him Ray, and everyone loved him. He grew up in Los Angeles, and I couldn't get enough of his stories about L.A. when it was surrounded by orange and lemon groves, about the Los Angeles River when it was more than a concrete ditch, about digging on the Santa Monica beach when the tiny grunion fish came ashore to spawn, about catching rattlesnakes by the tail in the hills of Redlands, and about being in *Lawrence of Arabia* when part of it was filmed in Hollywood. My father seemed to fill that vast California desert.

One day in June, Dad came home from his office hollering, "Aloooha!" as he usually did. At that moment I was sitting in a big plumeria tree in our front yard, watching a gecko stalk a

Check Out Receipt

Garden City Public Library
www.NotAQuietLibrary.org

Wednesday, March 8, 2017 1:51:13
PM

Item: 32001003618923
Title: On the dark side of the moon : a
journey toward recovery
Due: 04/05/2017

Total items: 1

Thank You!

fly. Geckos with the little suction pads on their feet that allow them to climb walls and windows were my current fascination. I felt woozy with the sweet fragrance of the plumeria flowers, the ones Hawaiians use to make leis.

"Aloha, my son!" he called when he saw me. "What are you doing in that tree?"

"Hanging out." I didn't want to tell him that I was just smelling the flowers and watching some dumb lizard. Nor did I want to incriminate myself by telling him that I'd spent the day on the Kamehameha coral reef at the edge of Pearl Harbor wielding a spear and killing things.

The Fort Kam reef offered endless exploration opportunities. At low tide, three of our gang had gone out there with a Hawaiian sling, a kid's version of a speargun, to poke at every hapless creature that stuck its head out of a coral hole: moray eels, octopi with their clouds of ink, stingrays, crabs, angelfish, and anything else that swam or crept between open ocean and dry land. Well, not quite anything; we avoided the man o' war, which had a nasty sting, and also the stunningly beautiful fish whose tail was a long lacy web that followed its body in seductive waves. Those "girly fish" we watched in awe.

Walking home from the reef we passed through a land of ambrosia: mango, coconut, guava, and breadfruit trees. The breadfruit looked like fresh-baked loaves dangling from a rope, inviting fools to temptation since they tasted like bitter raw potatoes. I swore that the tough green husks of coconuts could only be penetrated with a bazooka, but we soon broke them open by banging them on the street. Mangoes and guavas were pure sweetness. We scarfed them by the handful. Mynah birds by the score were an acceptable nuisance—they were loud and messy buggers, but we were sure we could communicate with them. "Hey, you bird, talk!" we'd yell. "Pieces of eight, pieces of eight, awk!" But those birds in the banyan trees never responded. There were also tiny birds with brilliant feathers—I recall red and green and yellow—that flashed from hibiscus to plumeria, carrying sunshine on their backs. But for me that plant called "sensitive grass," among the oddest of plants, with its unpretentious fronds that closed on your fingers at the lightest touch, was what most defined paradise and its sensual grasp.

The fact that a volcano was blowing up on the Big Island nearby seemed terribly romantic, in an adolescent sort of way. Not that I saw smoke or flames from the volcano, but I imagined them when I looked at pictures of Mauna Loa and Mauna Kea on the black and white TV. I saw still photos of the pahoehoe lava that was freshly laid down, smooth as black sand in an outgoing ocean. I learned about the a'a lava and its jumbled, sharp rocks. I knew the names of lava types just like I knew nearly everything about reptiles, or thought I did. I knew about sea snakes with their potent poison and the lizardesque tuatara, which is the sole remaining member of its order living on the islands off the North Island of New Zealand. I remember surfing at Eva Beach in Oahu—a paddle, stand up, fall, and do it again sort of thing—with my parents sitting impatiently on the beach or kicking around looking for seashells. Pictures of lava flows at Kilauea, on the ocean side of Mauna Loa, showed molten red rock oozing brilliant as fresh blood from a small crack in brown, drying pahoehoe lava. Another photo showed a river of flowing lava and viscous red daggers dripping down a stairstep on its way to the ocean. These images stuck in my mind like dreams of that flawless world; they were proof of the glamour and sorcery of events happening in the Hawaiian islands of my youth.

My father cleared his throat, snapping me back to the moment. "How was your day? What did you do?" he asked. A

KC135 flying tanker lingered in the sky like a big fat guppy floating down to the airstrip several miles distant. I was amazed that anything so enormous could stay aloft. The sound of its propellers nearly deafened me, so I jumped out of the tree to answer my father.

"Nothing much," I screamed over the noise of the plane. I was thinking that nothing I did ever amounted to much. He gave me a hug and stood back to study me at arm's length.

"Just looking at the flowers, eh? Very manly!"

"Well, not just that." I pointed to a head of coral that was sitting in a bucket of bleach looking like a big old cauliflower.

"What is it?"

"It's brain coral, Dad. I collected it for Mom out on the reef."

"That's nice."

"What did you do today, Dad?" I asked quickly, changing the subject. I didn't want to be cross-examined about hanging out with my friends on the reef, setting fires to cook what we speared, boiling crabs in a coffee tin, and blowing up stuff like the random hairspray can that floated in on the tide. There was something dangerous about the tide, but I liked it because it swept the reef clean. Every new day was pure on the reef, and what we did there was uniquely ours. All of us kids had sworn to keep these things top-secret. And we never thought about the hammerhead sharks that lurked around.

"Nothing much either. I worked with Northrop today. It's an aeronautics company."

"Oh."

We walked into the house together. "What's for dinner, Marj?" Dad said.

That was how our conversations went most days. Despite all the things we withheld from each other, I felt loved.

On the Dark Side of the Moon

I would have liked to ask my father about the war. That summer he took Mom and me to Saigon on a military "space available" basis. There was certainly plenty of space available to sprawl out on that plane at the time of what I now guess was part of the Tet Offensive, a surprise attack by the North Vietnamese on the city of Saigon. Our pilot landed in a nearly vertical pattern, diving down to the runway to avoid gunfire at the edge of the airstrip. My dad had business to do at the airport and he quickly left the plane. After we landed, airmen scurried around the airplane pushing large bags, formally, but quickly, into the cargo bay. Other airmen saluted each bag as it was laid into the belly of the plane.

I watched intensely as soldiers loaded the 6-foot bags. "Mom, what's in those bags?" I had a feeling. My mom leaned across me to see what was happening below us as I moved back from the small window. She saw what I did: the bags and saluting soldiers and the formality of their being laid gently into the plane.

"I don't know," she said. She looked shaken—she who was a navy medical technician in Tokyo after World War II—and held her silence for a long moment. "Maybe the bodies of dead soldiers, Mike." She moved away from the window and never again looked away from her book while we were on the ground. She didn't know what more to say about this gruesome reality of war, about the death of men who were drafted into carrying guns in a war that no one seemed to understand. But my head was pinned to the window.

The men were loaded one after another like sandbags that held back the rising tide of growing protests in the US. I remember some of the angry men getting R and R, "Rest and Recuperation" in Hawaii, getting haircuts, with their snipped hair dusting the barber shop floor as I walked by. One serviceman, disgusted by a song sung by John Wayne in support of the war in Vietnam screamed: "Fuck you, John Wayne! What the hell are we doing in Vietnam? It's goddamn crazy!" The barber shop fell silent, and the barber stopped cutting the man's hair, swept the barber's sheet off and said, "We're finished. Get out." He paused. "Get the hell out! Go." The soldier got out, casting a look at the other men in the shop who said nothing, and walked beside me. He said, "Hey kid. What's up?" I just stared at his half-haircut as he walked past. It all seemed so strange to me. I never understood any of that at my age—so I was told—but the men who rode in the belly of our plane that morning were all the reason I would ever need to oppose war. In those stacked-up bags I saw the decency and tragedy of lives, the killing that occurred without reason, the undeserved taking of lives, and sorrow. We did not have the eyes to see what we were doing to ourselves, much less to the hated enemy, the "gooks." There seemed no possibility of restoration.

When my father came back on the plane, little was said, although I pointed at the body bags that were now closed up in the hold. "We've got to fly," Dad said before I could speak, as he buckled down beside my mom. She gave him no notice. The plane went up like a rocket.

We changed planes somewhere and went on to Thailand, Taipei, and Japan. I always wanted to ask Dad, "What the hell were you thinking bringing us through Vietnam during the heat of war?" But I was too young. I can only imagine what my mother thought. I thought of the horror and the lesson of war that neither parent had seen through me. But indelible it was.

When we returned from our vacation in Southeast Asia, Dad agreed to help me make a skimboard as a Christmas gift. I wanted one to use when the surf was calm, and he said it would be easy to make from a piece of plywood: round the front and taper it to a squared-off tail, bevel the edges all around. Then I could shellac it. He thought a bullet shape would glide better across the skim of the outgoing surf than the round boards we'd seen other boys using. We talked about the cuts we needed to make on the board, then drew all of it out on a scrap of two-by-four. Finally we measured and drew lines on a sheet of five-eighths plywood.

The table saw whined and threw specks of sawdust as Dad and I ripped the plywood across it. He was a regular at the base woodshop, and he wanted to show his friends that his son could do this work.

"Now we'll spin the plywood like slo and run it back through on this sglin," he said. He adjusted his clear goggles and brushed sawdust off his flowered shirt.

"What, Dad?" My mind barefooted down the beach, along the sand of Waikiki, in front of the Polynesian Cultural Center. I startled tourists as I tossed the board down in front of me onto the glassy ebb of a broken wave just as it slipped back toward the ocean. I ran faster to keep up with the board, jumping on, hands in the air, riding it like a skipping-rock right into the next breaker, flipping head over heels into the surf. "Wahoo!" I imagined the shine and slide of the skimboard that was now only a dull piece of plywood in my father's hands.

"We've glot to rlun it black thloo." My father shook his head as if ridding his hair of a bug.

"What, Dad?" I gave him a puzzled look, but I couldn't hear much above the sound of the saw as he ran the board into the blade again.

"Now loo do't."

"What?"

"You mlake da next clut."

"That's funny." I forced a laugh.

"Whhhat?" His mouth moved slowly around the word.

"The way you're talking."

My father spun the board and motioned me to hold the edge so that the saw blade wouldn't bind. We ran it through again, splitting the line just right. Dad shut the saw off and adjusted the blade.

"We'll hlaff..." He paused. "Islge...." He paused again and looked at his hands as if they belonged to a stranger. He looked away from me, then flipped the switch back on. As he beveled the edge of the skimboard, the saw bound against the wood with a screech, stopped for an instant, then shot an arrow of plywood across the workroom. Everyone in the shop stared at the piece of wood as it bounced off the far wall and clattered to the floor. *"I'm slorry,"* Dad said very loudly in the direction of the shop steward. The steward smiled with tight lips, probably figuring that I had done the deed.

I had never seen my father make such a mistake with a saw. I noticed his whole body shake in one great shiver. He motioned to me with one hand to pick up the wood scraps and put them in the scrap bin. He put the unfinished skimboard under his right arm, dropped it, and struggled to pick it up. I shut down the saw as I'd been taught.

"Dad, are you drunk?" I had never seen my father drunk, but I had seen his buddy Colonel Cooper have a few too many at a cocktail party, and he sounded a lot like my father did now.

Dad's mouth made the shape of "no," but no sound came out. *"Nuuu,"* he said, too loudly. He grew silent for a moment. "Less glo, son." His eyes stared, and one pupil grew oddly larger than the other. My heart beat quickly as I picked up the skimboard, left the key for the table saw beside the stilled blade, and followed him quickly out the back door toward the parking lot.

"Dad, what's up?" Both of us climbed into the little black Mercedes that looked like an old derby hat and smelled of leather in a baseball glove. "What's wrong, Dad?"

He shrugged his shoulders and started the car, which lurched forward and stalled. He tried a second time and stalled it again. He pounded the steering wheel with his fists. "Yuuu must dlive."

"What?

"*Dllive.*"

"Drive?" I laughed awkwardly. "I don't know how to drive, Dad. I don't even have a learner's permit yet. Can't we get someone in the shop?" My mother once allowed me to practice driving in a parking lot, and I almost slammed into a streetlight. She had to yank on the emergency brake to stop us.

His jaw tensed; my dad closed his eyes and concentrated for a few painful seconds, as if conjuring the words. Then he spoke through clenched teeth. "Duh. Dlr. Drive! *Dlive us home.*"

I walked tentatively around the front of the car and got into the driver's side while my father slid over. I was embarrassed. We didn't live far away, maybe a mile. My father turned the key for me, and the car hummed. I had always wanted to drive the Mercedes, but now I was terrified by the prospect and confused by the circumstances. I waited.

"Plu da cla." Dad stomped to indicate the clutch, and I stretched my leg to depress it. He reached with his left arm and shifted the car into first gear. Breathing hard, he encouraged me to give it some gas by pumping his hand up and down, then motioned me to let up on the clutch. With a terrible grinding of gears, the car stalled. We went through the same motions again, stalled again, and Dad put his head on the mahogany dashboard. I thought he was angry at me. But on the third try, the car lurched forward and kept rolling. He clapped his left hand against the right hand in his lap and smiled triumphantly at me.

The night air felt sticky to me even with the trade wind blowing through open windows. I kept the car jerking along in first gear, rolling slowly around corners, through stop signs and a stoplight, steadily home through the heavy darkness. It was some kind of miracle.

***

Six months later, my friend Mike Fisher threw fastballs—nothing but fastballs—with pinpoint accuracy. "Fish" was my best friend, but he had already struck me out once already in this game and, anyway, I was angry at everything for no reason. He and I had bonded over our shared love for the Dodgers and our hatred for the Beatles; Koufax was "da kine," Maury Wills could steal any base he wanted, and the Beatles, well, they could go fly a kite. But this was another matter—a pressure situation: two outs in the bottom of the seventh inning, runners on first and third, my team down by two runs, and Fisher was a south-paw armed with sidearmed fastballs. I would swing for the fucking moon.

I picked up a handful of red Oahu dirt, tossed it down, and snuck a look at my parents behind the backstop. My mother had tied a chiffon scarf over her dark hair and rested an arm around my dad. She looked pretty and strong, a little like a Kennedy just then. My father had one arm in a sling and bandages on his head covering the smiles of stitchery where doctors had removed a tumor that caused his stroke. I was proud of them and embarrassed at the same time, and I couldn't make sense of the feeling. It was all so new to me. My invincible fa-

19

ther looking so like a war victim, and the new strength in my mother.

As I stepped into the batter's box, the coach signaled for me to bunt. Bunt? Hell, even with a good bunt the fielders could choose first or second for the final out or catch the runner if he went for home. Dimwit coach. When the pitch came hard and fast down the middle, I turned to bunt, but let the strike pass. On the second pitch, the coach still called for a bunt.

Fish held the runners on first and third with a look and threw me a watermelon, a big fat change-up like my buddy had never thrown me before: a gift. But on its way down the pike, the ball danced, the seams turning slowly like the edge of a continent on the hurtling earth. A knuckleball, but baby, oh baby, was it slow!

This pitch was destined for outer space. I took a hard, level swing that sent a line drive toward third base. The third base fielder just watched it sail. I rounded second before the left fielder even threw and kept going, past third, sprinting toward the catcher, who was now parked on home base like a hearse with the ball in his mitt, grinning.

I was out by a mile, and the coach benched me. I sat in the dugout watching my team toss a ball around the infield to warm up for the next inning. At least we were back in the game with a tie score.

"Muiiik."

It was my dad coming in behind the dugout. I could never tell how my father's words would come out. He was getting better and worse all at once. Sometimes he would cry unexpectedly, out of frustration, or regret, or I didn't know what. He couldn't speak. He couldn't write. He limped. Who was this man?

"Mliik."

I wouldn't look at him.

"*Milk!* He pressed his face to the chain-link diamonds. *"I'm your fal, you fa, fath-er."*

"I know. I don't wanna talk." I didn't want to hear his fumbling critique of the foolish play.

"Yes, *tak.*" He nodded his head vehemently.

I looked away and sat back pouting with my face in my glove. When I looked up again Dad was in the dugout, dragging me out. I was surprised by the strength of his good arm. He marched me away from the game and out behind the bleachers, where the ground was strewn with empty cups, Pixi Stix straws, and spat-out gum. He held my shoulders so that I had to face him.

"G'ood h'it, champ," he said.

I smirked. "Yeah, it was pretty good, wasn't it?

"Yeth." My father looked at me as if he was absorbing me, memorizing me for all time. "But you aim't Mlaurlie Willis." He smiled crookedly, one side of his mouth lively, the other drooping.

"That's Maury Wills, Dad."

He looked embarrassed, but he laughed. I felt bashful and foolish as he looked at me again for a long time. I wanted to watch the rest of the game. "You don't have to say anything, Dad."

"I *dloo*"

"What?"

"I *dooo.*" He looked around at the back of the bleachers as if he were a little lost. "More its… More than I can *slay.*"

"I know."

"You *dlon't know.*" He seemed angry. *"Shlut ulp, "slo* I can *tak.*"

I wanted to laugh at how funny that sounded, but his urgency stopped me. I looked at his tee-shirt with the word "Holokai" emblazoned across the front. It meant "walking on water" in Hawaiian, and it was the name of our 30-foot trimaran. He'd spent a lot of time on that boat sailing to Maui and Kauai, watching porpoises jump and flying fish smack the hulls. One time, I'd gone with him and some friends on a rough passage to the Big Island, the Molokai Channel. We all got sick.

My father, who knew so much about how the world worked—from war to law to skimboards—was sinking before my eyes. I knew exactly what he was going to say, and I didn't want him to. I wanted to maintain the partnership of silence. Words were the enemy, and somehow the silence meant nothing bad could happen. I did not want to hear my father say "I love you," even if it was the one group of words he never screwed up. He leaned toward me and looked me directly in the eye. "Son, I am going to die soon."

I felt a hard ache in my stomach. "No you're not, Dad." It was a knuckleball that I didn't know how to hit. "You're not going to die!" I put my arms around him and held him close.

"There is nothing we can do about it, son."

I closed my eyes and held on to my father, and we rocked side to side as if we were sailing together, slapping over the rough ocean through the Molokai Channel. I couldn't come up with any words except "I love you, Dad." We held each other for a long time with the trade wind carrying the smell of the ocean to us on the red-dirt baseball diamond.

Chapter Two

Confabulations

Thirty-two years melted away when I saw a vision of a figure coming out of the mist. In a flash, I wanted life again. I called out, "Kah-to, Ree-ta." Was I hallucinating? He heard me. "Kf-tah." The figure moved toward me. It was Doug. "Fu-fat." Thank God! He's here! I'm saved! He heard my grunts and found me.

Doug came over to me and stopped short. He called for Katie and Miguel. Most of the blood all over my face had dried, and one side drooped like the jowls of a basset hound. I had been there for roughly four hours while they searched for me. They searched in a line, side by side in the rugged lava, and planned to give it up in half an hour, when darkness would fall. Only by luck had they found me in the dying light of the ruby sunset.

My body hung in an awkward question mark, with my good arm hugging the branch with all the strength I had. Doug could see I had fallen oddly, and he didn't want to move me. He thought I'd broken my neck. Finally the three of them decided to move me very carefully to a level and grassier place. Then Katie went off in a hurry for help.

I desperately wanted water. Doug looked at me and fell silent, believing that water was the wrong thing to give me. He walked away to smoke a cigarette and collect his thoughts. I recall his smoking vividly; Doug was no smoker. Miguel gave me a cup of yogurt, which I opened all over myself with one hand. It was subsistence. I passed out, came back, and hummed to stay awake at Doug's insistence.

After an eternity of semi-conscious singing, I heard the tremendous whir of propellers as a helicopter touched down nearby like an enormous dragonfly. It had taken Katie three hours to cross the kipuka, make a phone call, and come back with a group of rescuers. When I talked with her afterward, she said she was frantic. She'd taken a wrong turn, gone 35 miles in the wrong direction, and was almost out of gas. But she'd made it.

The flashlights of rescuers winked like fireflies as they came toward me, slowly, like ghosts gliding across the dark and broken lava. When they reached me, one of them put a scarf over my face as if I were dead. They put me on a stretcher, carried me to the helicopter, and loaded me like 160 pounds of hamburger. It had been nearly seven surreal hours since I had fallen in Craters of the Moon.

The helicopter took off, grasshopper-quick, into darkness. I tried to sit up. The kind nurse said, "Just relax. It'll be about an hour." I was a wounded man now. I was shot in Korea or Vietnam or Iraq or Idaho; it didn't matter. I was broken, and I remembered corpses being loaded into our plane, the deafening sounds of a flying tanker as I climbed down from a plumeria tree to talk with my father. It was delirium. The helicopter flew on through the unknown blackness back across the Great Rift, until we finally landed at a hospital in Pocatello, eighty miles southeast of where we'd started out in the lava.

Two men ran to the whining helicopter, put me on a gurney, and wheeled me lickity-split into a hospital bed under brilliant lights. Masked technicians loomed over me. One of them cut off my favorite yellow storm jacket and my tattered blue jeans while another shone a light into my eyes. A third scanned me for broken bones with an X-ray machine. People in gowns took my blood pressure, recorded my pulse, and the number of respirations per minute. They put me into a contraption that produced a computer tomography scan of my head, showing an area inside that had died, a place in my brain where a clot blocked an artery, making a dark, still pool of blood that took away life-giving oxygen.

An orderly wheeled me into a culvert-shaped machine, one I later came to recognize as a magnetic resonance imaging device. He said, "Hold still so your brain can be photographed with radio frequency." I grunted to confirm that I'd heard. The orderly pushed a button and a conveyor belt fed me into the hollow soul of the machine, which began a mad dog growl and whirling sound. When it had its fill, the orderly wheeled me from room to room and put me through more and more procedures. All I could see were the masks of concerned nurses and doctors who leaned into the bright lights above me. All I knew was that these strangers were caring for me through my endless nightmare.

I woke the next day with intravenous tubes carrying liquids into me. I could barely move and I couldn't speak. When I tried to roll over, it dawned on me that I couldn't move at all on one side. A doctor appeared and held my hand. "Mike, can you hear me?" I nodded. He looked directly into my eyes and spoke with enormous sympathy. "I'm afraid you're paralyzed in your right limbs." I closed my eyes. Paralyzed, my ass, I wanted to tell him, but I just gurgled and felt nothing but terror and terrible loss. Then my mother came from out of nowhere and was informed by a doctor that I might have had a brain tumor. My mother? What was she doing here? She lived in Sacramento. Brain tumor? That was my dad's malady, not mine. But I couldn't tell her that as she held my hand gently.

All the nurses and doctors in their clean, white clothes came to care for me and tend to my every need, most of which I couldn't understand. Seeking to define the dimensions of my tragedy, they came to poke me and check my reactions, to question me and look closely at my infirmity--questions I couldn't answer, and reactions I didn't have. They wrote on clipboards and vanished, coming and going like mists on the lava.

A team of doctors wheeled me to another room and bade me swallow something. It was a command performance, and I just had to trust them when I signed with an X on the permission form. The lights suddenly went out, darkness squeezed in on me, and when the lights came back on, a doctor pulled his mask off and said: "Mike! Mike, can you hear me?" I nodded feebly. "Mike, you've had a stroke, but there is no heart damage from the clot. Do you understand?" I nodded once again but I didn't understand. I'd had a stroke that killed part of my brain, but at least I wouldn't die from a heart attack. Some consolation. I had come perilously close to dying out on the lava. Somehow I survived. Maybe it was the doctors' work on me, or maybe it was my soul's decision on the lava; I couldn't say. Now I'd taken a gift of life, but why didn't it seem much of a gift at all?

In attempting to protect Idaho's wild landscape I had almost killed myself. Now I would have to rehabilitate my body and my mind if I had any hope of helping rehabilitate this land I loved. Everything that mattered to me--thinking, writing, loving, working to protect Craters of the Moon--had vanished. I couldn't know the magnitude of the struggle before me, nor the energy it would take to come back from this stroke. Unraveling my confusion, recapturing what I had lost, would be measured in geologic time.

During those first days in the hospital, dozens of friends visited. They came from Ketchum, Boise, Challis, Salt Lake City, and California. It was remarkable to me. But I remember only snippets of their visits. I talked incessantly, but quickly I saw that nobody could understand what I said. Doug, Miguel, and Katie were the first to visit, but I didn't recognize them and don't remember their presence. They were told to leave by doctors. Scott and Christie, friends from Salt Lake City, talked closely at my face and passed notes that were unintelligible because I couldn't read a thing, but I remember their attempts to communicate with me. Scott and I had worked closely together in Utah to maintain Utah's wilderness. Their compassion astounded me and Christie was full of caring and love. Jackie and Ralph, from Pocatello, floated above my head and seemed to come and go for no reason but sweetness. Bouquets of flowers came from everywhere, it seemed, and dozens of cards and letters arrived in the first two weeks. My mother stood beside my bed taking in all of this support.

In a week I was able to begin, tentatively, walking, with a deep limp. What a gift it is for paralysis to fade away and movement to become possible! One time, my friend Renee drove from Boise to visit me. She insisted that we go outdoors into the spring sunlight, so I rolled in a wheelchair out to a nearby football field, where I managed to ask Renee to dance. She laughed uncomfortably and said, "How? You won't fall, will you?" I said, "May-be," with a smile. I got the volunteer caretaker to help me stand and I held one arm out to Renee. She grabbed it and we danced, or anyway we didn't fall. It wasn't an elegant maneuver, but it felt like magic to me. A few days later I walked with Bill and Sara, lawyers and good friends from

Boise, who stayed for an afternoon and brought food and kindness. My recovery seemed to be proceeding at a rapid pace as the swelling in my brain went down, and I felt encouraged. Fortunately, my mom put dozens of cards and letters into two big notebooks where I could see them and know that I had caring friends and, of course, remember all of them.

Merritt Frey came to visit from Washington, D.C. I'd met her at a conference on water quality problems in 1998 when she was working for the Clean Water Network and I worked at cleaning up Idaho's water quality for ICL. We corresponded when we got back home and I agreed to meet her at the Peery Hotel in Salt Lake City the spring of 1999. I wanted to take her to the southern Utah desert, which I knew from my days with The Wilderness Society. We spent a nice evening getting to know each other again at the hotel bar and a passionate night in bed. The next morning, we left for southern Utah with a decidedly blissful glow. We hiked down Fish and Owl canyons near Blanding, basking in the shade of a vast cottonwood tree, and swam together in a plunge pool below a delicate waterfall. The trip was over much too soon. On the way back to Salt Lake City we argued about road conditions, directions, and control of the car, all of which seemed odd to me. But Merritt was lovely and we worked out our differences and moved on together. By Christmas of that year, Washington, D.C. seemed way too far away. When I had the stroke a few months after, she flew to Idaho immediately to be with me. It wasn't so far away at all.

I didn't want Merritt or any of my friends to see me in my diminished condition, but I did want to let them know I was fine. Of course, since I had entirely lost the ability to talk intelligently, to write, and to walk normally, I wasn't fine. I couldn't think straight, but I knew that I was loved and all that love would be one of the greatest reasons to recover. I was determined to be what I had been before, which was, after all, only two weeks from what I was today. But when my friends left the room and Merritt went hiking near Pocatello one day, I cried buckets of tears in frustration. All right, I would fix myself as soon as I could, no later than the middle of May, I figured. If I could walk already, it would be no great effort to talk and think clearly.

On April 20, as I lay in the hospital, a woman came to my bedside to give me physical therapy. I didn't know I needed any. She got me up from the bed and introduced herself with a bright smile, took my hand, and walked me very slowly to the bathroom, because my limp remained profound. Her name was Susan, she said, and I found her enchanting. She was young, and I remember that she showed a lot of perfect teeth when she smiled. Susan moved her hand to shake mine on my left and I grabbed it. It was a reflex, nothing that I had thought out, and it surprised me. Her hand in my hand: that is yours, this is mine; self and other. These were new concepts.

Susan picked up a leather pouch and brought it into the bathroom. She put it in front of me, and I looked at it dumbly. She reached into it and handed me an object.

I took it-a black, vaguely familiar plastic object. Something to scrub my teeth? After all, this was a bathroom, which was where I usually brushed my teeth. I raised it and began to rub it across my teeth. Susan smiled. "No, that's a comb. You use that for your hair." She spoke so sweetly, so kindly.

Okay, yeah, of course, it's a comb. A comb, right. I felt fire in my cheeks. Jesus Christ, what had happened to me? My hair. That's on my head. I rubbed the comb flat on my head. Got it.

"That's it," Susan said. She pulled something else out of the pouch like a magician. What next?

"That's a toothbrush," she said, and held it out so I could clearly see what it was. I nodded, not betraying what I was thinking: *what, exactly, is a toothbrush?* But mostly I thought how gorgeous her long red hair was and how interesting her face. I wanted to ignore what I couldn't say or think. I stared blankly at her.

"Do you know what to do with it?" she asked, speaking as if to a child.

No, apparently I didn't, not exactly, though I'd had a vague recollection just a moment ago. How depressing it was not to know a comb from a toothbrush. She rubbed a finger on her teeth to show me.

"Teee," I said blandly, and motioned to my face, aping her. This was childish stuff. Why couldn't I make her understand?

"What is it?" she persisted.

I didn't know what to say. I repeated, "Teee." But the truth was that I didn't know the first thing about this object that I had seen every day for 44 years.

"Yes, that's a toothbrush."

"Yeth, that'sa I, uh, wha…"

She pulled a flashcard of a toothbrush from some other magic place and held it out for me to name it. She covered the name, and I couldn't figure it out. I made a motion of rubbing it on my teeth. It was just a guess. When she uncovered the name, I could read it. "Tootbrus," I said with difficulty. I felt like a fool before this younger woman, and I didn't want to let her down. But if I could barely name a toothbrush, what did that say for my ability to explain the finer points of my job, to insist on control of overgrazing practices, ORV abuse, and vandalism in Craters of the Moon National Monument?

Confabulations

As the days went by, I imagined my mother crying outside the door of my hospital room, but I never saw her tears. I was now utterly dependent upon her. I did recognize her and a few of my friends, doctors, and nurses, but all I said was "Mmmm" as I nodded to them. I couldn't remember their names. Mom--I got that one. Her name was Marj. I felt like a thing to be observed, fed, watered, and cared for by relatives and friends— a burden. I was now unable to command my circumstances, which was what I had done, fiercely, before the stroke. I was a grown man with feelings and perceptions that I had lived with for 44 years, but I had lost them. Where were they? Overnight they had been replaced by only the faintest impressions of what had been my life. I missed my life and had to work to regain every bit of it, piece by piece.

In late April, I was released from the Pocatello hospital, and I had hopes that things would change, that I would soon go to my office and continue working for American Lands, an environmental organization with its main office in Washington, D.C., and an outpost in Idaho. I was glad to be headed back to Boise, my home, to figure out this near-death catastrophe. I felt ecstatic to be out of the hospital, but it had been weeks now, and I was not healing as quickly as I expected.

My life moved in slow motion while the rest of the world zipped around. I was a koala in a leopard's world. I felt vulnerable, barely alive, and I missed the sparkle that I felt had defined me. I expected the miracle of immediate healing and understanding. In time, I learned that roughly one-third of those who suffer a stroke die from it. One in five must be institutionalized. Another 40 percent have some permanent impairment. Not exactly good odds—only one in 15 comes out of a stroke totally untouched. My walking, though, was coming back as if it were ordained by God. It was nothing short of a biblical recovery, but I didn't recognize that; I was selfish. I only asked: *why did this happen to me?*

Everything looked oddly brand-new as Merritt drove me and my mother home to Boise from the hospital. Had Merritt come again, or had she been here all along like Mom? Maybe she'd taken a really long hike. I wasn't sure how long I'd been in the hospital; a week seemed like months, a day like weeks. All that I saw became real only moment by moment. Merritt lived a long way from Idaho. I knew she was the woman I had a relationship with, but I really didn't know her at all. Why had she come here? Just to drive me from Pocatello to Boise? I liked seeing Merritt in this role as a compassionate woman. It was odd to see my mother and my girlfriend together, which seemed a perilous combination at best, since both had very particular ways of doing things.

I climbed into the back seat with some difficulty, dragging my slow right leg. My right arm lay on my belly in a sling and was of no use; I had to lug it around as I pieced my past together again. I imagined myself as my father, with a bad arm and a tendency to cry as he looked across the expansive lawn of Tripler Army Medical Center.

Pocatello is a dry town on a flat, where trees grow only as long as they're watered and supported by a thread of irrigation water. But the hills in the foreground glowed green as we drove along, and behind them the tawny color of last year's grass was still on the mountains. In the higher mountains beyond the hills, a single line of cornices tucked into the shade, was melting into small, shining streams. In front, grasses blew in a wave of golden hair. That made me giddy, and I laughed out of joy for the beauty of these mountains, and just for the way life turns out. All of this world is so fragile, so gorgeous, so very perfect and illusional.

Confabulations

Inside Merritt's rental car, objects were new toys to be touched and understood. What was the thing that shot out the cool air? "Marj, could we turn on the air conditioning?" Merritt had asked, as Mom slipped a CD in the player. I puzzled over the CD playing songs, the power windows rolling up by themselves. Right, it was the air conditioner that cooled air, but how was it conditioned? I was fascinated by all these things and each of the words that described them. I thought I had never seen such marvelous things or heard such miraculous words. The automobile seemed a beast that we controlled, its internal power roaring at the turn of a key, coming alive and carrying us off, away from Pocatello, away from this unfortunate, unforgettable town where the hospital lay.

I saw lines of trees beside the Holt Arena at Idaho State University, so many students and so much green, green grass as we drove out of Pocatello. The students were fresh and alive; everything brimmed with springtime. I felt it, too, but the students were in a different world, becoming educated adults, while I was starting kindergarten and learning life all over again.

My mother turned and looked at me. "Mike, what's so funny?"

I could only spit out random words: "Mou-nta-ins... grass... me-lt" and a hundred bits of gibberish.

"Yes," she said, "that's funny." She responded to my laughter even though she couldn't understand me. But that didn't matter, because I knew she supported me. I looked at the ceiling of the car and wished she could read my mind, or I hers. I couldn't speak my mind, so I kept silent. Instead, I offered a smile, a smile that would serve me in this world of confusion for a very long while. A genuine smile that said: "No problems."

On the Dark Side of the Moon

We accelerated on the freeway, with fences flying by and cows wandering behind the fences. The car kept going faster and faster, a hundred miles an hour, two hundred, a thousand, too fast for a numb mind. A dumb mind. Fence posts flew. It was the fences that kept the cows away from the freeway. Or the cars that kept the fences from hitting the cows. Or they separated each other. I liked the cows, was fascinated by the cows. They were mooing or bellowing, eating grass. And what was the grass? Cheatgrass! Cheatgrass was a name I recalled. A short grass, ten inches at the seed head, trident-shaped heads that weren't very nutritious. That's what it was, cheatgrass. What an interesting word for the universal weed that dominated so much of this landscape—it was poison, it cheated. A poison brought here by cowboys, for cows. A poison that was spreading and reducing wildlife habitat on millions of acres of the West. Okay, that was what I'd known. Now I knew it again, just by seeing the land as it passed. I hated the cows, didn't I? Accursed bovines! They moved swiftly past.

After a few miles, I noticed some big metal wheels connected to round pipes that sent silvery, shining solder far out into the air. I could hear them faintly, even with the air conditioning on. Chink, chink, chink, chink, they sounded, as the silvery substance kept flying out in bursts. Water was the fluid--of course it was water--water shining in the sunlight, with pressure forcing it in a line that moved steadily until a small paddle interrupted the flow—chink, chink, chink, chink. Sprinklers, water pressure—suddenly I knew they were called sprinklers. Speech may be a discrete skill in the mind, but speaking in my mind didn't help me pronounce a word out loud. Nor did I remember the word for long after saying it and seeing it in my mind. I remembered traces of the word, broken like ripples fading in a reflecting pool.

Confabulations

What causes water pressure? The water came out like it was brand-new and eager to spurt: magnificent and beautiful, the silver lines running out for a hundred, two hundred feet and dying, shining on the grass like dew, like tangled kite strings, pretty as shining gossamers. Everything seemed like a game of chess, and all this half-knowledge made me crave more knowledge. It was out there, in there, in my brain, emerging not in a linear fashion but chink by chink by chink.

In my brain, the thought suddenly connected to the sight: irrigation. Oh, yeah! It became clear: the Snake River, its dams and canals like arteries, with pumps and sprinklers, the siphon tubes that were moved by farmhands. This paraphernalia moved water from the river to the crops in small bits. It was a visual image, a snapshot, that stuck in my mind more than any precise memory. This was a short history of the Snake River as it was irrigated and lost to the fields. In my mind, all this history, this learning, came back in the tick of a few seconds, almost as dreams come out of unconscious imagery. Unconscious images had been learned by repetition over many years, it seemed, but I had to absorb these images consciously and work to remember them. The flow of the Snake River was how many CFS? That was an odd thought, but somehow I knew a CFS was one cubic feet per second of water.

I pointed at a machine digging up the land and tried to make Merritt say the word. "Oh yeah, it's springtime, the tractors are plowing up the soil," she said, offhand. My love for Merritt came and went like a tide in the ocean, and now I felt sad and happy and grateful to need her and her most offhand knowledge.

"Trak-ter," I said, trying to hold the word as the image and the image as the word. Everything became a clue to something I already knew. Springtime. Tractor. Plowing. Soil. All these concrete words seemed to fit, to be familiar, but only when I saw or heard them in their context. My vocabulary seemed brand new to me, but they were my same old words, my old, comfortable thoughts. I had much to regain!

Further on, I saw long, tall willows dancing and swaying, churning in the wind, looking like trees in a van Gogh painting that I'd seen somewhere. They seemed to blow and burn and flow with a pure, powerful energy, an essence, a spirited being-ness, lightning in the soul. But after a third look, I saw only the arrow-shaped Lombardy poplars. Their radiance now extinguished, they were just trees, mindless, inanimate, blowing in the wind. Or were they? The same thing happened a month later, when the shivering leaves of aspen and cottonwood trees gently rained upon me in Ketchum. These slender ghostly spirits seemed to lay their hands on my head and impart a powerful healing influence. Then I watched them turn back into what they were, and what had been was gone: blown up, blown together by logic.

A part of my altered state of being seemed to have been put out like a candle flame, and I was a little more in the world of the real, the concrete, and the rational. What an exquisite pity it seemed, however, at once to see and to lose the wonder, the poignancy, the raw magic and muscular power of nature. But once seen and felt, I know that these powers exist, whether they ever occur again; they are within.

When we got to Boise, we piled out of the car at the house I had bought just the year before, in 1999. I had had big plans for improving in the new millenium. Now my Mom, Merritt, and I spoke of the little jobs I could do, things like putting dinner in the oven or turning on the heat so as not to freeze. They seemed trivial, but it turned out that most of what I could do was sleep, eat, and watch TV. Merritt had to go back to D.C.

and her job, and I was lonely for her, but I tried to stay upbeat for my initial appointment with Dr. Weiss, a neurologist in Boise.

My mother and my longtime friend John McCarthy, whom I'd helped hire for the Idaho Conservation League many years back, came with me to the meeting with Dr. Weiss. It all went well, as far as I could tell, until the doctor asked me about my family history. I told him about my three children in my broken language. There was a strange silence in the room.

"Mike, you don't have three children," my mother said incredulously.

"I, uh, don't? No. Unh, no. I guess I, hmmm, I, uh, don't, do I?" I felt jolted by uncertainty. "Ow many?"

"None."

"No, I doln't ha, hal any, do I?"

"No, unless you've been holding out on me."

We all laughed uncomfortably. I'd have to remember that next time--no kids. I was asked about my father's death many years ago. Is he? Yes, that's right. I knew that, I said. And I did. I fidgeted, expecting to be corrected at any time about the facts of my life. What was this awful torture? Let it be over! I knew I had made a big mistake.

"Octor, ow m-m-much am I goin to reagain?"

"What, Mike."

"Re-again? Re-gain?"

"I can't say."

"Why no?"

"Well, the brain works in odd ways," he said, with what I thought was a sympathetic look. These were strange words from a medical doctor It sounded as if my brain were some deity. It wasn't. It was mine, and I was in charge of my brain. "I can't say how much damage there has been," Dr. Weiss went on. "Your story about your children tells me that there's still some swelling in your brain. It will go down. I'm sure it will. I know that's not you. That was only a temporary confabulation; a fantasy." He paused and looked directly at me. "Why did you tell me that?"

"I don kn-ow. It wa-wah-as wa the firs ting that pop p-ed in my mine, my mind" I felt like Lewis Carroll's Alice after she reads the poem "Jabberwocky." Alice said, "Somehow it seems to fill my head with ideas. Only I don't exactly know what they are!" This astonishment like Alice's, had carried me through the looking glass into a world most bizarre. I didn't know right from left, black from white. My brain was a bowl of oatmeal and I felt Alice's alarm: Then it really has happened, after all! And now, who am I? I will remember, if I can! I'm determined to do it!' But being determined didn't help her very much, and all she could say, after a great deal of puzzling, was 'L, I know it begins with L.'"

I knew the objects that words described, but I couldn't say the words and had to search for them in my mind. For instance, if "house" was the word I'd lost--as one time it was--that could lead to a world of mistakes. I knew what a house was. I lived in one, smelled its dustiness, smelled the new paint and the garden in back, and surely I must be paying the mortgage. I knew my house, although I couldn't say that it was my "house." Without the right word, life became a scavenger hunt, a minefield of misunderstandings.

Before the stroke I had always been able to come up with the right word when I needed it. I had been a writer, a speaker, an environmentalist paid to sway opinions. When I said the wrong word for my house, I called it a "hut." Well, as Mark Twain said, "the difference between the right word and the almost right word is really a large matter—it's the difference between the lightning bug and the lightning." My inappropriate word led to a variety of guessing games before we got to the word "house." We did manage to get a couple of guests into my small castle, however.

Sometime during the next blurred month, my friend Belinda came over with cookies. Sweet, charming, and mischievous Belinda with sweet, charming ginger cookies. As we sat talking in my living room, she paused for an awkward moment, which was unusual for her, and then blurted out, "Mike, can you get a stiffy?" Her voice went up an octave--it became her mother's voice--when she said the word "stiffy." Silence reigned while I thought about it.

Belinda was a good friend, but not someone I would ever have expected to ask me outright about the condition of my penis. I slowly ate a sharp flavored cookie as I considered her question. It seemed that everything led to sex somehow--jokes, the way women dress, the way men dress, our demeanor, the cars we choose, the way we speak, and walk and act—so it was a natural question and probably an important one. She just wanted to know.

I was embarrassed, but I muttered, "Well, uhm, yes, yes I do." I thought I did, but I wasn't sure at all, to be honest. I just couldn't say that, and the thought of never having sex again worried me enormously. But there were other things on my mind with the craziness of the stroke.

However, I'd heard that people who have had strokes had a hard time having sex. I had to find out if I could get an erection. So when I got into bed that night, I turned off the light and masturbated, half-fearful that this stimulation would trigger another stroke. But so be it. My penis got stiff and I kept rubbing it harder and harder until that familiar ecstasy ran over me. Never had an orgasm been so joyous, so rewarding, and so complete, with every nerve of my body alive, tingling, and, more than anything else, working. The semen made a celebration on my chest as I let it run wild, dribbling down my side until it dried in a crust. Never had I been so proud of my own body to respond so forcefully and so happily to this fundamental phenomenon. I was quite simply astonished to retain this gift and smiled about it all of the next day.

I went to the internet to find out if others experiencing a stroke had somewhat the same experience. Doctor Jose Vega, a researcher and stroke specialist at Columbia University, writes that a "…stroke is almost never a direct cause of sexual dysfunction." Dr. Vega adds that fear of having another stroke, the depression associated with a stroke, and the immobility caused by the stroke can cause some people to stop having sex for a period of time. He also mentioned a few very rare circumstances where a patient's genitals become numb or their sex drive suffers. I felt grateful, enormously grateful, to know that I could be pleased by sex and share that joy with my lover.

A few days later, I told Belinda that it felt pretty damned good just to swell up and squirt. She laughed and said "Wanna share, Mr. Medberry?"

"Maybe not, but you can imagine," I said.

***

If I had to experience the pain of re-learning my own language as if I were a child, I was at least blessed to see what had been given me to lose. I had spent a lifetime ignoring or taking for granted small things like bees or butterflies, which now seemed to offer great LSD-like wisdom. I had a new sense of meaning that redefined my perspective on life, like the first view of earth from outer space. I felt the vibrancy of being a child in an adult's body, the sense of growing up again from helplessness to mobility, from silence to speech, from mindlessness to mindful thought.

Still, I needed an outlet for my anger about all that had happened. There was a doghouse in my yard, a kind of Byzantine castle made of hardboard and two-by-fours on a bed of what was now rotten wood. It had everything but a moat. Whoever built it had shingled the roof—now invaded by yellowjackets-- and fortified the whole thing with chicken wire, staples, and nails. It was a doghouse to last for the centuries. It was also a perfect place for my anger, and I wanted it obliterated so that I could plant flowers in its place.

Over the following month, my anger became an all-consuming fury. Week one: I tore off one wall of the doghouse. It must have weighed 150 pounds, but it was still attached to the structure by chicken wire that unraveled into a big, nasty mess. I freed it with a hammer, tin snips, and fury, then dragged it to a trash heap, cursing. But the work taxed me, and I had to sleep and salve the merciless stings of the goddamn yellowjackets. I felt weak and rested—literally—for days, and then came at it again.

Week two: I took down another wall of the doghouse after half a day of fighting it and drinking tea in the hot sun. Two walls down, two to go, plus the roof. I couldn't believe this fucking thing was built as solid as the Berlin Wall. *But fall it would!* I promised myself.

Week three: Tear down this wall, Mr. President. Tear it down! It must have been there for twenty years, thirty, forty; it was my age. And its roof was re-shingled when my house's was. Down with an axe, down with a sledgehammer, down with a maul, down, down, down. Somebody really loved his damn dog to have built this goddamn thing. I kept whaling at the doghouse until I pounded my thumb and let out a cataract of swear words.

One of the odd tricks played on my warped brain was the way I could still remember and unleash every cuss word that I'd ever known, and maybe a few new ones that I hadn't. It felt good to swear out loud in the daylight. I took on the two standing sides of the doghouse in a rage and brought them down in a thudding crash, along with the accursed roof. Finally, the deed was done, and I burned the doghouse to a smoldering rubble. I rubbed my sore thumb—my left--and realized that I'd used my right hand, as I'd done before the stroke. Satisfaction, and my life can move forward. Now I could plant roses, apple, and apricot trees in the restored garden.

***

Surely, I told myself, the Elks Rehabilitation Hospital in Boise would agree to take me in soon, once they were assured that the swelling in my brain had gone down and I was able to learn. During the eternity of the next week, I met with therapists, doctors, social workers, and nurses about what they called my "brain attack." They deliberated about what to do with me as I tried to go back to work. I went into my American Lands office and tried in vain to reply to hundreds of emails and dozens of answering machine messages. I struggled in vain to remember my password on the recalcitrant computer. I tried hopelessly to talk with key environmental contacts whose names I found in my address book. I labored cluelessly to organize the papers on my desk. Each effort ended in disaster. I left my office in tears.

The grass greened around my home, but my soul was badly bruised. I had to sleep fourteen or fifteen hours a day. I could barely put one thought after another. At times, I couldn't even remember what to eat, and I cried out of frustration about nearly everything when no one could see. I felt guilty about keeping the American Lands job when I couldn't function, make decisions, or set policies for the organization as I had in the past. American Lands had chosen to keep me on at good pay that I no longer deserved. Realizing that their generosity was driving them to poverty, I quit the job I loved.

Instead, I found a job as a janitor in an architectural firm. It wasn't much, but it paid me for doing something I could understand: wipe away dust on the desks, wipe down the counters, suck the dirt off the floors with a vacuum cleaner, mop away the stains. In one office, there was a photo of a determined woman racing on her bicycle, and another of fellow bicyclists with their arms around her cheering a victory. I found out that she was an Olympic competitor and she eventually won a gold medal. And who was I? I had the love of my friends and my mother. That love, it turned out, counts for much, and it was what I held on to in bleak days. Love gave me strength to identify what I had lost and to work on regaining those qualities. But I was still lost and purposeless.

What was I doing? Nothing. I often felt lonely and dispirited. I slept and doddered in my backyard. I thought. And forgot. I cried over my losses and worried about my future. I waited for my brain to heal, waited for therapy like some drug, wandered the hillsides near my house and waited for my mind to fill in holes and complete itself. I could feel myself getting better, but slowly, ever so slowly, as if I were rediscovering syllable by syllable the language and land of my past. But that past seemed to hold little future.

My mom moved into my house to be with me until I could cope with the outside world. She went back to Sacramento once a week for the first couple of months in an effort to sell her house there and make arrangements to move to Boise. In my house, she made curtains for each window, gave me quality furniture, paid most of my outstanding bills, and left notes with phone numbers for me in case of emergencies. She made dinners or bought takeout for the two of us. She put together two scrapbooks full of cards and comments from my friends. She was also sensitive to my need for privacy when other people came to visit. She didn't want to be a prying mother, and she moved out of my house in another month to a house one block away, having created a safe place for me to live.

Mom had raised me alone following my father's death when I was 12. We moved from Los Angeles to Sacramento, when Los Angeles was a smoggy and dangerous place. By the time I left home at 17, I needed breathing room, so I went to the University of California in Davis. After I was at college for a couple years, my mom suggested that we go to the Bay Area every other month to see a performance. She loved the theater and wanted to reconnect with me. We did that for about a year, and I gradually came to know her as the fine person she had always been. After I graduated and moved to the near-wilderness in McCall, Idaho, she came to visit me. I was 25 and in the process of building my third house, the first in Idaho, just outside of town. Her visit was a disaster. It ended with accusations of drug use and poor judgment when she read my journal. It was all true enough, and well-documented, I might add. But we never patched up the breach that erupted between my poor judgment and hers at reading my private journal. Only 20 years later, after my stroke, did we forgive one another. We had each learned our lesson, and when I fell on my face in Craters of the Moon, it was good to know that my mother was there to help me up. I hope that I will be able to return the favor if the time comes.

Confabulations

I thought a lot about Merritt. I'd known in January that her being in Washington and me in Idaho precluded our having a meaningful love. It was fun, but it couldn't amount to anything substantial. We talked about this during the winter of 1999, but now I was badly impaired with a stroke; I was damaged goods, and she was so much younger and more vital than me. Still, she'd shown no signs of pulling away, and I couldn't help wondering how she might fit into the confusion of my house and yard. Maybe we'd put in a garden with more fruit trees, solar panels, and a new bedroom. We'd replace the carpet and paint the walls. On a good day we'd be compatible.

I had occasion enough to sit around in my doghouse-free backyard. One day I chose to write in my journal about what I saw. My scribblings were filled with egregious grammatical mistakes and misspellings, but just the fact that I could write at all was a home run. Here is what I wrote:

I saw a bug and could not name it. Why should I fight with its name? Why fight with any name at all? I watched it land on a leaf, brilliant green leaves on a bush. It did not hold or withhold anything; it spread out its wings, gracefully, slowly opened and closed them. I observed its bars of yellow, painted with solid black lines defining the yellow patches, these quivering rods with tiny, solid balls on top, and the beady black eyes, surprising patches of bright blue and orange stripes on its shoulders.

I watched as it unrolled its tiny thin black straw of a tongue and tested the leaf. Dabble. Dabble. Dabble. Apparently it had no luck. The creature flew to another group of leaves in the same bush, but in flying it swooped widely and glided elegantly before me. It flew like I imagine a magic carpet flies, stalling with its wings on a cushion of air and easing down to a stop, then dancing up and fluttering. It shined with an iridescent glow in the sun which turned yellow and blue as it landed on the bush

45

again. The bug set lightly: four wings, hair on the blades; a small black creature wearing a big yellow cloak lined with black stitching. I knew that thing! What was its name?

I moved my hand to see if I could measure if it was four or six inches upon my finger. Closer to four. No, stay! It flew in a dreamy flight, a dalliance with the sun. The sun now on its back. What was that? This was one of my favorites. A tiger! An insect. A swallow-tailed. A tiger-tailed swallow. Nearly. A Tiger Swallowtail butterfly! A Tiger Swallowtail butterfly. I named it!

Chapter Three

Healing My Soul

O n May Day, 2000, less than a month after the stroke, I tried to write a letter explaining my compromised condition to a literary agent. I had been searching for months for an agent to represent my new manuscript of short stories to publishers, and just before the stroke I thought I'd found one. After focusing my thoughts, I sat down and began to write.

~~Dade~~ Deard Ms ~~Mi M M~~ Wales
I ~~hog~~ think have been a at much ~~tonin tomines~~ monie
At ~~deuniz hou tDoug TOW tephimes decaping~~. I ~~serehd & tvor~~
I ~~would toce~~ I ~~would~~ would ~~sulfilx~~
Surly ~~tou~~ and.
Eliz I can occure your

I was trying to tell her that I'd had an accident but would get back to her as soon as I could. But I couldn't organize my thoughts. Not even close. I couldn't figure out if what I'd written was connected to what I meant. How could I ever communicate with an agent about my writing, or with anyone about anything, with a mind so totally crashed? On May 9, I wrote another piece of a letter in my journal after I had given up my immediate attempts to contact Ms. Wales.

> Oh, well hay about?
> What about this? I wonder ~~wou woulder whae~~ would.
> I really wonderd ~~wihous~~ Good
> Gold I just forbord adoud this. How as I come
> To take a tack take ab
> A schared? How will ever
> Take anon thourt?
> Oh is my. Oh is my!

I knew I was making progress when I compared the two versions of my writing that were separated by a week, but it wasn't much progress. I closed my journal with the letter I'd begun the week before and stared out the window. What the hell was I going to do? The goddamn window was covered with dirt spots and cobwebs, and I wanted to throw a dictionary through it. I knew the general idea of what I wanted to express, but I couldn't write it. I sat on the couch and put my face in my hands.

What had I *not* lost? Everything in my life was catawampus. Had Merritt come for a visit just last week, or was it back in April? Had she gone home and come back and left again? Where was my mom—California, or was she here? I was cogent for moments and opaque for the rest of the day. Or the week. I was afraid to feel hopeful when I regained something, because it was soon lost. I was an inchworm on a treadmill, gaining inches on a marathon run, when I moved forward at all.

I remember talking with a friend one afternoon on the broken steps of my back deck. He asked what I was experiencing, and in my hallucinogenic haze I told him that the pieces of my brain were a blizzard of blowing pages ripped from a book, cast to the wind, scattered like confetti or tickertape, with all the little letters falling down one by one. I had lost the organizing principles that allowed me to give order to my thoughts and my world. My memory was all broken paragraphs, broken sentences, broken words, or simply blank. There was no order, no path from A to Z. My brain had been covered in a cloak of night, and I could see only pinpricks of stars to give me a bearing. The conductor of the symphony had walked out of the building, and the players warmed up in a familiar way, but they played no symphony whatsoever. My mind was a riot of mixed metaphors.

I asked my friend how I could begin pulling the pieces together. My house had always been full of stacks of paper, a mess, true, but a mess I knew I could dig into and find what I needed. Now I was utterly baffled just looking at the piles. My friend understood piles of paper; I knew his work habits were as messy as mine, and I respected him for all that he did. I knew he was a wise man, and I meant to get some advice from him. He shook his head with the utmost sympathy and smiled. "I'm sorry, Mike. I don't understand what you're saying."

I looked at him blankly. What could I say that would have meaning? It seemed that I would have to pick up the letters in my mind, recognize them one by one, imagine them and lay them on a piece of paper as if I were playing a cosmic game of Scrabble with myself. Form words, then put together sentences, then paragraphs, then pages of paragraphs, then begin to order the pages in some mindful, meaningful way. Communication was a game for two or more, and for now I couldn't play. I needed some logical handhold, some point of reference, to lead me to what I had previously done by instinct. This was a puzzle of time, memory, and intelligent thought. Piece by piece, I had to solve it in my mind--time and place in a logical sequence and then to integrate the context in the real world to communicate. It would have been easy to give up on solving this complicated puzzle, but surrender simply wasn't an option.

For months after my stroke, I couldn't retain most things that were not written down. I couldn't write worth a damn and my speech came out garbled. I held on to the conviction that knowledge would eventually come leaking in to my conscious-ness and that these piles of random information would once again have meaning. *Have faith!* I told myself. My brain was ob-viously not the tool it had been, though. It was damaged, but it was what I had at the moment on this weird, wandering jour-ney toward knowingness. At stake was making sense of this world that I had lived in for forty-four years. This world had disappeared like light from a shooting star.

There must be a way out of this conundrum, and to learn a new but familiar way of being. *Know thyself, Mike. Take time to re-learn who in the world you are.* It was the simplest and oldest ad-vice. And the hardest to follow.

I felt that Merritt loved me for the person I was. She had come to Idaho when I was a wreck, but just before that I dis-counted her as living too far away and had begun to see another woman. That was a short-lived relationship that couldn't en-dure the stroke. Merritt came to Idaho twice to accompany me in my darkest times and offered me encouragement and con-versation. We planted a small garden together where the dog-house had been and walked through my neighborhood looking at and naming the local plants and grasses. We rode our bikes together after I learned to ride a bicycle again. Once, she came with me to my office and tried to help me get me back to work. She made me feel comfortable as I remembered the fundamental tasks of living. She made me laugh when I made silly mistakes in speaking. She wanted me to heal and fly again.

When Merritt was growing up in Michigan she'd had an accident in which her horse fell on top of her. She was nearly killed and her parents tended to her after finding her with a crushed pelvis. She had worked for months, years really, to recover and to this day she walks with a slight limp. Despite all that had happened, she retained a great love for her horse, the animal that nearly killed her. This was what I loved about Merritt: her capacity to recover from a tragic event and still to feel fondness for the horse that created her disability. But it also told me that she was stubborn and ardent to recover what she had lost. She was a woman whom I wanted to spend my time with.

My mother offered all I could ask of her. She bought a house near mine and sold hers near Sacramento, a remarkable sign of her unconditional love for her only child. We had moved from Hawaii to Los Angeles after my father's death and lived in their old house, and then we moved to Sacramento in 1970, into a house by the American River. Sacramento provided a peaceful place to grow up surrounded by hop fields, vacant lots and levees beside a river that was oh-so American. And oh-so my mom.

One day in early summer, when she thought I was able and interested, Mom suggested that we take a roadtrip in Idaho. "Where should we go?" she asked.

"Ow bout Craters? I would like that." I felt like Humpty Dumpty. I had taken a great fall and had to put together the pieces of this broken egg: confidence, communication, love, sanity, work, and memories. And all of it related to Craters of the Moon, where I had fallen and lain out on the lava for many hours. This was a harrowing memory, made more poignant by the time-sensitive ischemic stroke that had permanently damaged my brain. I say that my stroke was time-sensitive because doctors give stroke victims three hours to get the person to a hospital to treat him with a clot-busting medicine, before lack of oxygen kills the afflicted cells. It must have taken me 8 hours to get to the hospital in Pocatello. We never spoke of this, but it reminded me just how precious time can be. I wanted to confront this fear and show my mother the beauty of Craters of the Moon, which I had worked to protect over the years.

"Yes, that would be a good place to go. I haven't seen it yet, and I know you love Craters of the Moon. I'll bring Tika along." Tika was a tough 15-gallon barrel of a dog, a cattle dog who was Mom's constant companion.

"It'll b' hot," I said. Mom offered to drive, and I suggested that we stay in the one-buggy-town of Carey. My driver's license had been suspended after the stroke, but I got it back by passing a driving test while I was still unable to speak clearly to the examiner in Boise. I pointed when she asked me where I was going and shook my head when I should've said no. I smiled gratefully when she said I had passed. Still, I was relieved when my mother said she'd drive. By nightfall we found a cheap motel in Carey, and I was fast asleep when the door was nearly bashed down.

"Jenny, let me in!" came the drunken voice at our door.

"Get lost!" Mom said in her toughest, lowest voice. "Go away!" I was definitely awake now. My mother's voice always became lower when she felt afraid.

"Come on, let me in!" The door was thin as cardboard.

"There is no Jenny here," Mom growled. A bare lightbulb glared starkly as she pulled a string above the bed.

"Oh come on, let me in," he pleaded. More pounding.

"Get lost!" Mom parted the curtains and peered out the window.

"Mike, he's just sitting there," she whispered tremulously.

"He'll go," I said. But he didn't.

"Get the hell out of here," Mom bellowed, "or I'll call the police." Tika started barking wildly.

"No!"

"Then I'll call the police." She spoke in an even deeper voice, as the little Australian cattle dog continued her piercing barks.

There was silence from outside the door for a moment. "Ok, ok," he muttered. "Jesus." We heard his thudding footsteps recede.

"Now let's get some sleep," my mother said as she pulled the light string.

I had done nothing to get rid of him because I felt I couldn't speak well. I'd left it to my mother, and I felt like a coward. Lying in bed, I was eager for daylight.

As I lay there tossing and turning, I thought about my mother's courage. It had served her all of her life, through growing up in the poverty of central California during the Great Depression, while serving as a medical technician in Japan after World War II, having a hysterectomy in a lonely hospital in Washington, D.C., losing her husband to a stroke and brain cancer, then almost losing her son in a similar way--and maybe, most of all, through being raped in her youth.

These were things that my mother never forgot, although she didn't often bring them up. They defined for me who she was, and why she lived with compassion and fear, understanding and joy. We talked about her life now and then over the years when we were driving somewhere together, and in Boise when we had time. When I asked her why she never remarried she replied, "No one ever asked me after your father died." And that was that. Of course, it wasn't; she's an attractive woman and everyone gets lonely, but it was a closed question. I know this much, however: she wanted the best for me, and that was why she moved to Boise. I felt her love and tried to return it.

In the morning, Mom asked what we should see in Craters. She had outlived the night and was ready to go again. Over breakfast we pulled out a map, and I suggested we drive the 7-mile loop road from the visitor center. From there, we would take a short hike. I wanted to prove that I could still make my way and show my mother that I was not a useless son. I offered to drive.

I drove half the loop and parked at the southern end. I proposed that we walk toward a group of tree molds which had retained the shape and texture of the tree trunks that were incinerated by flaming lava 2,000 years earlier. I pointed out a well-defined trail, but my mother wanted to stay in the car. "It's hotter than hell," she said, "and the place looks awfully desolate. It looks like the Sahara. Tika and I will turn on the air conditioning and wait for you. Don't go very far."

I set off on my own, examining minuscule purple flowers and feeling the rough path through my boots. After half a mile or so, I turned around, afraid of triggering another stroke. I headed back to the car, where my mother was waiting and worrying. I told her that I had looked out across the boundary of the national monument and imagined expanding this protected territory to bring in much of the surrounding land. This hike seemed, she said, the first step on a thousand-mile journey.

I found that navigating accurately with a compass was no problem for me even in the anonymous expanse of lava. That came as a surprise, because a doctor warned me that my sense of direction might have been obliterated by the stroke. He told me not to go out wandering alone. But what would my future be if I couldn't find my way along a simple trail? I had to be able to figure out where I was in a landscape, because I had always loved finding deserted, empty stretches on long runs and hikes. Now I was confident that I could find my way around and get back, even if only on a short route. That was enough for now. I could read and follow a map. I could identify places to go, and places that were important to avoid.

We stopped often to look at the landscape along the seven-mile road. The terrain of tortured chunks of basalt in the lava flow reminded me of bodies being stretched like taffy in the heat of melting rock. In another place along the road, a football field-sized expanse of cinders the color of burnt sienna had fallen a thousand years ago when a cindercone blew up nearby, or so said a National Park monument sign. We parked and both of us walked out into the field of tiny cinders which were as light as popcorn. They made squeaking sounds under our feet. Little grew in these queer places except the white webs of a few pioneering plants. Tall cindercones, looking like large piles of black sand, stood against the 11,000-foot Pioneer Mountains in the background, a drama of severe contrasts that shifted under creeping shadows of clouds. Long grasses swayed on the faraway mountains, conveying motion that echoed the sweep of time. In the foreground, tiny, brilliant magenta monkeyflowers and balls of dwarf buckwheat bobbed in the wind. This stillness and beauty had prevailed for millennia, bringing awe and peace to those who beheld the scene. My mother and I walked along in silence but for the squeaking of cinders underfoot.

A well-worn trail just off the road, ascended Infernal Cone and brought us to a panoramic view of the receding land. I took a quick trip to the summit by myself, and from the top I saw flows of lava in shades of gray and black, the darker lava marking more recent and rugged flows with patterns cutting the jigsaw relief of the land. Big Southern Butte rose abruptly from the Snake River plain 10 miles north, and gave additional dimension to this piebald view. Behind it, Borah Peak rose to more than 12,000 feet amid the high Lost River Range in twisted cirques and ridges. In the farther distance, the Teton Mountains seemed small and faint, a pointy, incongruous alpine setting, crowning the vastness of closer, coarser lava flows. I drank in the view and climbed back down to the car, and we drove on a couple of miles to where the Caves Trail began.

I had wanted to see the caves in Craters since I first read about them, 12 years ago, in a 1924 *National Geographic* article by Robert Limbert. Limbert, a part-time explorer and writer, earlier was one of the first to map out this eerie landscape of lava, over a pair of expeditions in 1920 and 1921. A lively storyteller, gunslinger, and all-around flamboyant character, he popularized the name Craters of the Moon and championed protection of the area until President Coolidge designated the original 54,400-acre national monument in 1924. Limbert's *National Geographic* article was part of his public relations campaign. His descriptions of his marathon journeys caught my imagination, though I had to admit the way that he died—of a stroke—made me shiver. At least he wasn't hiking in Craters of the Moon at the time.

Mom wanted to stay in the car with her stout little dog. It was a short hike from the car to Boy Scout Cave, so I went alone. That cave comprised a dark, cramped tunnel opening onto a natural ice rink that a young skater could glide around with room to spare, or so said a second *National Geographic* article. I saw only a shrunken pad of ice that would tempt none but readers of that article to bring a pair of skates along. It disappointed me. The enormous Indian Tunnel, a quarter of a mile away, descended as a gash into the ground. As I walked in, light shone in oblique cracks, splashed like quicksilver on the floor. It dazzled me.

The Devil's Orchard, near the parking spot where I began, was a befuddling cluster of tall demonic basalt structures that had been carried along on flowing lava. Juniper trees, redolent of gin, grew in hollows and humps of ground beside the dancing devil's den. Pahoehoe lava dried in the form of pythons coiling around each other, daring me to walk on their backs to make a shortcut. In 45 minutes I was back at the car with my mother and Tika.

"How was it?" Mom asked. Tika panted.

"I feel re newed."

From the end of a spur road jutting off the loop near Buffalo Cave and Broken Top mountain, we could see part of the Craters of the Moon Wilderness, created by the passage of the Wilderness Act of 1964. The Prairie stretched out as far as the eye could see, and I understood why this kipuka was named The Prairie. It is a lovely, shabby, shrubby, grassy area dotted with pyramidal buttes and cones, but it is surrounded by lava. It was a glorious place to be, and I felt it calling to me when my mother and I turned to leave.

On the way back to the visitor center, we saw pure black lava and large cracked blocks that looked like Volkswagens left out in a rock junkyard beside the road. We passed the Blue Dragon lava flow, with its unique, iridescent glow that is created by a film of titanium left on the surface of the rock as molten lava cooled. This landscape is as weird and unknown, as numbing and spectacular as tundra on the North Slope of the Brooks Range in Alaska, in which I've hiked; it is similarly arduous for hikers moving across hummocks of melting land as across a'a lava to make progress.

My mother drove us out of the monument, across the duo-tone lava toward Ketchum, and onward to the distant, developed landscape of Boise. Back home, we rested after our long, strange journey.

"Did you enjoy it? Was it pretty?" she asked.

"Yeh, kinda," I replied. "Da wak was go-od." Then the conversation drifted, and we talked about California and all our relatives and friends who lived there. However, my mother and I never talked about long past arguments between us and all the things that had separated us for so many years. The angry comments we'd made to one another, the painful things we'd done--these petty things were done; they had vanished. I was chastened by the stroke, and now the past didn't matter at all.

Out of the blue my mother said, "Mike, you're my son. I would do anything to help you." I was silent. She had come to Pocatello, then to Boise, had given me beautiful furniture for my house, had sewn the curtains, and helped arrange the financing for the house. And what had I done to deserve that kindness? At length I said, "I love you, mom." The words came out all right, and we took another step on that thousand-mile journey.

***

While I slept that night, I dreamed of neurons racing around in my brain, randomly at first, until they found each other, connecting neuron to neuron. Then, once enough of them had formed into clusters, a light grew in the room that had remained dreary for months. The light sparked, glittered, turned red, brightened, then a pure white light made the room glow as if the sun shone through its windows. In an adjacent room and then another, new lights popped on, until every room was lit and my house was full of brightness. The weak neurons grew connections until they all formed around the injury from the stroke. I thought them through the maze to their partners. In my dream, I consciously prepared myself for the challenge I anticipated the next day when I would have my first appointment with Lynae Nielson, my primary therapist at the Elks Hospital. I decided that every neuron would be lit and every thought would be clear for the meeting with Lynae.

Lynae is an enthusiastic and discerning woman. I didn't like her at first because she was strictly business. "Say this," she directed, bidding me to watch how she formed the words with her tongue, lips, and mouth. She told me to fill in the imaginary blank: "A cat walks, a fish ___." I didn't quite know the difference between a fish and a cat. For all I knew, this fish could fly. I knew it should have been obvious. It wasn't.

The breadth of my ignorance loomed as Lynae pushed me through this and similar elementary tasks. They showed me the precise degree of my loss. I felt darkness in my soul and was embarrassed and humiliated by the exposure of my weakness. But as I worked through my depression I recovered what should have been obvious. This was the only way to get better: to feel pain and frustration like a child growing up, and to push through it. Lynae understood. I had to get beyond the distractions and self-indulgent complaints and be willing to dive face-first into my own brain-mush. I made it clear to Lynae that I wanted to regain every single thing I had lost in April of 2000. When I thought about turning away from the arduous path before me and not reaching that goal—well, it was unthinkable.

Even though I had my license back, I did a lot more walking than driving those first months after the stroke. When Merritt came to visit in June, we walked all over the east side of town. She helped me recover the names of the trees and flowers that were blooming around us as we climbed the Boise Foothills one evening.

"What are these?" she asked me.

"White flowers."

"Oh? What kind?"

"Pre-tty."

"Yes."

"Sy."

"It's a sy tree?"

"No, sy-ringe."

"Like a flu shot?"

"No, no." I shook my head vigorously. "Syringa."

"Oh, syringa. That's the name of it?"

I nodded.

"It's a beautiful plant," she said. "It smells good!"

Merritt was gorgeous, and I was a wizened old man; she was kind, and I was a speechless curmudgeon. She didn't know the trees and flowers of Idaho, but I was able to teach her these things as I groped for their names. She was East and Midwest, and I was a Westerner through and through, but we were both conservationists, and we filled each other's voids. We watched darkness crawl across the city and felt at peace. I told myself that she was way too young for me and wondered why she felt good with me. We enjoyed in each other's company and felt the incomprehensible grace of love.

During her visit, Merritt and I went for a mountain bike ride, taking a shortcut that I hoped would allow us some privacy. Well, it did, though the steep climbs and rocky slides nearly killed both of us. We got home bramble-cut, exhausted, muddy and a little amazed that we made it back at all, but we laughed about it. The next day, Merritt hopped in a taxi and flew back to D.C., and I missed her immediately.

Healing My Soul

Inspired by her visit, I threw myself back into my work at the Elks Hospital. Lynae and I agreed on a plan of attack covering seven categories: receptive language, expressive language, reading, writing, speech, cognitive skills, and organizing skills. To regain what I once had, I would first have to master each of these diverse yet interconnected skills. This was key: we were going back to the familiar terrain of my experience. The experiences existed somewhere in my brain but we had to extract them. As a team, we entered the raging wildness in my brain and worked to reconstruct how I expressed myself and defined the building blocks of understanding and communication. Lynae helped and prodded me all the way, gently but incessantly.

Receptive language skills were the ability to receive a singular piece of information and know what it meant in a larger context. For example, when someone said, "How are you?" I should be able to respond by saying "Fine, thank you." I couldn't do that when I first came to the Elks Hospital. This simple phrase was part of the reality I had lost, and it slowly occurred to me that this was more than a mere convention: I had to demonstrate that I understood the question and each response had to make sense. In essence, it should be more than a mere rote response. I remembered my second-grade teacher telling me to write the following one hundred times to punish me: "Learn to listen, and listen to learn." The phrase stuck with me, if only for the alliteration, but that was my task once again.

Expressive language skills meant my ability to express myself in speech using proper language. At stake was making myself understood. Obviously these were critical skills. I relearned how to state my name, address, birthday, education, and occupation. But I often omitted the words between nouns--verbs, adverbs, adjectives, conjunctions—which proved exasperating and confusing for those trying to understand me.

On the Dark Side of the Moon

Some of my worst experiences involved phone calls where I had to parlay with an automated system.

"Hel-lo," said a mechanical voice one day. "Thank you for calling U.S. Bank. This call may be monitored. Please choose one of the following options: press one to hear your account balance, two to make a payment, three to report a lost credit card, or four to repeat this message." For some reason, I panicked and pushed two on my telephone pad though I meant to hit one.

"Please provide your personal identification number." My what? Oh, yeah, my PIN. I didn't remember it, so I waited for the message to end. I got flustered and just pressed one.

"Please wait while your call is answered. The approximate wait time will be...five minutes." Slam! I hung up and redialed.

"Your call cannot be completed as dialed. Please hang up and..." Oops. Slam! Redial.

"Hel-lo. Thank you for calling U.S. Bank. This call may be monitored. Please choose one of the following options: press one to receive your account balance..." I pressed one.

"Hel-lo. Thank you for calling U.S Bank. Please enter the last four digits of your social security number, followed by the pound sign."

Let's see, that was 7112. For God's sake, I remembered it! That made me feel exceptional.

"Please enter your account number followed by the pound sign." Not a clue. I had no piece of paper with my account number on it. Shit. Ah, my checkbook! I found it on the dining room table and punched in the number.

"A representative will be with you in...seven minutes." I planned what I would say as I waited what felt like a century.

"Hallo, may I help you?"

"Yes. I'd uh, liketohave my, uh, account number."

"Your number? That's the number you dialed in, sir."

"Yes, uh, the money I uh, have."

"Your money?"

"My balance."

"One moment, please." She went off with a click and returned with a hurried voice. "Please repeat your account number, sir."

I chuckled at being called "sir." "I don't, uh, know where is it. Just a min--"

"I'm sorry, please call back when you have located the account number. Thank you." Click.

"Shit! You worthless, assh--." I would try it again tomorrow, with both of the numbers I needed written down beside the phone. What else would go wrong? However, the next day I nailed it. I felt good accomplishing this essential yet utterly annoying task.

On the other hand, I found most of the words I wanted when I talked to my friends. I corrected my mistakes by backing up and trying again, just like repeatedly backing into a parallel parking spot. Sometimes it worked, sometimes it didn't but eventually it always did. Sometimes my friends would respond with a polite pause that allowed me to correct myself. Or else they might say the apparent word for which I was reaching in silence, and our conversation moved on. Lynae had told me that most people don't listen for perfection in conversation; they just want to communicate and share ideas that interest them. No one noticed my stumbling; it was simply static on the radio. Why sweat the small stuff? No reason except my pride, and pride still affected my self-confidence and achievement.

Lynae similarly broke the act of reading into its constituent parts, and my skill progressed over time on a middle path between writing and speaking. First, I matched words and sentences to pictures to show her that I understood them. Then I recognized words and rehearsed their meaning one at a time, word by word. A few months later, I could read sentences and explain what I read, which meant that both my speaking and my memory were improving. Lynae would have me read paragraphs and quiz me about their content.

"Mike, what does this mean?" she asked one day. "Would you read it?" She laid a newspaper on the table before us.

"I don't know, exactly." I looked closely at it. She pointed to a headline: "Babbitt Says Craters Expansion Likely."

"Oh, it means we're winning," I said.

Lynae laughed. "I guess that's true. You are. You've got those sentences right. Now read the first paragraph." She pointed to it, and I read it out loud in broken speech. It was great news!

According to the *Idaho Statesman,* Secretary Babbitt had recommended that President Clinton expand Craters of the Moon National Monument by 737,000 acres of land. There would be several hearings on the proposal, but the President apparently had the blueprint for protecting three quarters of a million acres! The monument expansion would ensure that the Bureau of Land Management and National Park Service portions of this divided land would begin to heal together. But for the dogged determination Robert Limbert had shown more than half a century earlier, and the work of many people unrecognized in the meantime, this proposal to expand the monument beyond the original 54,400 acres would not have been possible.

There was nothing sudden about Babbitt's proposal. It had been moving as surely as a rising tide from the time Limbert lobbied for a larger national park proposal for Craters of the Moon in the 1920s and settled for the smaller 54,400-acre national monument. In 1964, Congress and the President designated the Craters of the Moon Wilderness, and in the 1970s federal law established Wilderness Study Areas on the BLM land. The Idaho Conservation League, Congressman Richard Stallings, and the University of Idaho had all offered significant proposals in the 1980s for Craters of the Moon. But Babbitt's proposal was the biggest plan for this region, and it needed the support of President Clinton. The prospect came as a shock to conservative Idaho Republicans.

Though I was immensely cheered by the news, the *Statesman* article also reminded me of how little I could do to affect the fate of the expansion. After so many years of working to protect Idaho lands, I had become a silent observer. Still, as Lynae implied, Babbitt's provisional victory paralleled my own tentative win over the stroke. Both of us were making progress, but the challenge was barely half over.

In a few more weeks, I was able to attempt a novel again. Lynae assigned me a chapter from *The Mapmaker,* author Frank Slaughter's fictionalized account of the 15th century venetian cartographer Andrea Bianco, which I read as homework and then summarized for her the following day. I had to read each chapter two or three times to understand it and follow the plot. It took me about a month to finish and at times it felt as though the book itself was a guidepost to understanding. Within another three months, my reading skills passed muster with Lynae. She understood I *could* read now, and I would. And I did: *Lying Awake, The Wonderful Wizard of Oz, My Year Off, The Diving Bell and the Butterfly,* and *The Decameron* to name a few. Two of them, *My Year Off* and *The Diving Bell and the Butterfly,* are memoirs written by stroke sufferers.

Recovery was slow, but it also seemed that I lived a decade in ten months, gaining what time had cost me 10 years to learn the first time, cost me only a fraction the second. I gained renewed appreciation of the remarkable joy to be found through reading, as well as astonishment at the process of reading. There was nothing quite like relearning everything I already knew to refresh my sense of wonder. The writings of John Donne, Emily Dickinson, Anton Chekhov, Edward Abbey, Flannery O'Connor, Jorge Borges, Franz Kafka and dozens of others were now alive in a way I hadn't expected. I learned to read again the way a child does: letter by letter, word by word, sentence by sentence, chapter by chapter, and book by book.

Emboldened by my success as a reader, I began writing more. I gave a friend of mine, a professor and writer, a piece of writing that I wanted him to critique, half expecting a glowing commentary. Instead he wrote back to me: "This is a difficult sequence to talk about for two fairly obvious reasons: 1. The fact that you're trying to bring together two essentially different subjects, your stroke and the environmental case for protecting areas such as the Craters of the Moon National Monument... 2. The stroke itself, in particular its resulting and continuing verbal disabilities, which, I'm sorry to have to say, do show up here in the handling of language and sentence structure."

I was devastated, but a pound of truth was what I'd asked for. It felt more like a ton of critique, but it was gently offered. Like everything else, my writing wasn't what it had been. I would have to work harder to fix the holes in it. And there were many. I would have to think harder about the process of presenting and constructing ideas clearly. God knows writing had never been an easy task for me to begin with. I started attending writing conferences in Idaho and California, were I blundered my way through the workshops at Squaw Valley. I offended people and shamed myself, but also made a few good friends. I read books on writing: Annie Lamott's *Bird by Bird* and William Zinsser's *On Writing Well,* among others. I felt as if I was working on my master's in fiction writing for the second time, a student again, but alone now, as I struggled to understand the mysteries of writing. I went over and over my work: five versions, seven versions, and more. I edited until I thought one chapter, the first in this book, was marginally acceptable. Wonder of wonders, my favorite magazine, *High Country News* and editor Ray Ring agreed to feature the story, and later *Black Canyon Quarterly* published another version of it with the support of editor Kate Wright. It felt good to be writing again!

Speech, however, continued to plague me. It presented a problem that never went away, as the stroke had made a direct hit on this skill. There are thousands of component parts making up the act of speaking, like delicate gears in a complicated watch. When I opened my mouth, they went haywire, knocking into one another, springs flying everywhere in a flurry of exotic sounds.

"Now push your tongue against the pressure," Lynae said, holding a wood palate on my tongue. "Practice that." She drilled me on words and phrases, tongue-twisters like "devastatingly delicious delicacies," "fresh fruit float," "bleached black blouse," which featured consonant clusters I had the most trouble with. The more slowly I spoke, the better I sounded. I made an effort to control the rate of my speaking so that I enunciated words more clearly. This discipline turned out to benefit me in many ways. Slow speakers seem to think about what they say, making them precise, like a capable newscaster. Although I didn't like being forced to slow down, I realized that I should have done it years earlier. Before my stroke, I tended to outspeak my colleagues; now I learned to listen to them. It took a stroke to show me that most people actually had pretty damned good thoughts if I could shut up for a moment to consider them.

But all of the speech and listening skills in the world couldn't get me *thinking* as if I had never had a stroke. The most debilitating of the cognitive problems I faced was the continued failing of my short-term memory, or "working memory." I could barely remember a mouthful of words as I spoke them, much less commit them to my long-term memory. Somehow I remembered the words I had known for years, but I couldn't remember the pattern in which to place them as I spoke. It was a long time before I could remember what I said yesterday, an hour earlier, or even 15 minutes ago. What I said or heard was lost unless I made a concerted effort to write it down, reread it and repeat it, until I had committed the pattern to my memory.

"Working memory" is much like the random access memory in a computer. Imagine a computer with no RAM—no auto-save, no saved files at all, nothing in its memory bank for long-term retrieval. Such a machine would continue doing the same task over and over because it had no way of remembering what it had just done. I had lost significant parts of my RAM. I paused every six or ten seconds, after nearly every sentence, to think about what I had said and the next thing I wanted to say. I spoke tentatively because I was never sure exactly where I was heading, which in turn undermined my confidence in my judgment. I lost track of what I was saying mid-sentence and had to pause to collect my thoughts. Spontaneity? Hell, forget it. Spontaneity is that verbal ability to make random connections quickly and seemingly naturally in a way that pleases and startles listeners. I had always been good at such clever remarks. Now I could no longer be witty--a part of me I would forever miss. Quick thinking was what I had always offered to lighten up critical judgments and get my opponents to laugh. Now all I did was repeat everything, and that made me a sitting duck.

I had to accept such compromises in my life even as I gained ground. No longer could I craft perfectly clear policies to define a victory, nor could I mold the executive decisions required to create conservation plans for an enormous wilderness proposal. There were also a number of victories.

At the Elks Hospital I had an occupational therapist, a woman named Kari Smith, who was kind and understanding without coddling me. She taught me organizational skills like balancing my checkbook, using my daily planner, buying groceries, and baking cookies--all things I had forgotten how to do.

Kari had me write out a shopping list of items I planned to use for dinner: flour, sugar, baking powder, chocolate chips, nuts, and vegetables. She handed me a wad of money, counting it in front of me as I tried to concentrate.

"That's a good list of items," she said. "Now let's go to the store and buy them."

Kari drove us to Albertsons where we danced through the electric entrance doors. It was summer, and the Fourth of July was only a week past. The store was still decorated with American flags. Kari smiled and directed me to a shopping cart. I was overwhelmed by this bumper-car world and the subtle barriers that guided us into the vegetable section. I stared at the orange, yellow, and red bell peppers. "Ok, good, Mike," she said, her brisk steps matching her determined nature. "Let's pick out some vegetables and get some baking ingredients." I felt as excited as a Labrador puppy.

"Ok," I said. I wondered at all the people who were buying vegetables, taking one here and one there so easily. How did they choose? I picked up an apple, then three apples, thinking:

pie. I could almost taste them, my mouth watered—cinnamon and sugar, delicious, tart, green apples!

"What will you do with the apples?" Kari asked patiently.

I thought for a moment and smiled like a 10 year old kid. "Eat 'em."

"Well, ok. But think about the money you have, and your task."

Thinking about it was fine, but counting the money? I couldn't. The shiny green apples held my attention: the rich color soothed my eyes; in my imagination their sweet taste made my mouth water, the pressure of my teeth on their skin became a seductive longing, the flesh a firm, popping feel in my mouth, the cold, tart juice squirting onto my lips, dribbling down my chin. Reluctantly I put the fat, gorgeous apples back on the fruit table. I couldn't remember when I had last eaten an apple. I would return here where apples lay in endless bounty, where apples begged me to eat them as if for free, where their freshness would taste like all that was sweet and sharp and pleasing; I would get good and sticky and satisfy myself fully. Another time.

I grabbed red and orange peppers which were on my list. But there was a cut watermelon beckoning under cellophane, green on the outside, sumptuous red under its hide, defining perfect beauty: juicy-looking, sweet-smelling, the mouthwateringly red flesh rising around black seeds, alluring and tempting. "Let see, what doowe need?" I said as we walked to the baking section of the store three aisles away, but I still was thinking about that watermelon. I imagined the sweetness of it, the thirst-quenching power, the red and black and green of it, the beauty and the metaphor in fruit: creating an image and then tasting it in my mind. I had been a literal man ever since the stroke and this sudden casting off the mere factual made me shiver with gratitude. If imagination could return, maybe humor and spontaneity would, too.

"Check the list," Kari suggested.

"Oh, uh yea-h, list." I had slipped it into the breast pocket of my shirt.

"How about sugar?" she hinted.

"Okay, sugg-ar, four uh, flour, baking powder, choco-late chips, nuts. Ok." I put these things in the shopping cart and we headed out through the traffic of other carts and shoppers. I wanted to honk my horn as we waited, and then, suddenly, all the things I had gathered were in opaque plastic bags. I paid for the groceries with a ten and a five. The checker took the bills and gave me change, which I pocketed without counting. "Thank you," I said.

"You're welcome." She smiled brightly. She had no clue about what I'd learned in coming to the store, finding food, and giving her the cash. I learned that confidence lay in believing that everything would work out fine—regardless of the facts or my doubts--and by simply acting as if it were true. But regaining my imagination and the power of metaphor was the greater victory for me.

We drove back to the Elks Hospital, and Kari set me up in the kitchen near her office. I got to work baking cookies: setting the oven, measuring out the ingredients, and using the proper utensils to mix them. When Kari left for a few minutes, I swirled the wooden spoon into the dry ingredients, added water, and slurped a taste of the batter. It was silky, with a few bumps of unmixed powders and tasted bland, bittersweet, and soothing in a way that only chocolate chip cookie batter can.

"How's it coming?" Kari said, peeking in to check on me.

"Oh, umnh, fine." I didn't think she'd caught me with a spoon in my mouth—unless she was watching on a hidden camera. I still had to bake the cookies, clean up, and put away everything I'd used. My timing was a bit off, but each of these activities proved an indelible learning experience, reminding me of what I used to do.

Kari left again and I finished my job. The cookies came out thin and wrinkled.

"Mike," Kari said. Her voice startled me when she returned. "We need to count your change and return the balance to the till."

I had stuffed the change in my pants pockets. Now I dug into the pockets and dumped coins and paper on the counter. The coins rolled everywhere. I counted the bills: "Fife, six, seven, in cash." I put them in the till and started picking up coins. "One, two, three,…"

"Those are dimes," she said, pointing.

"Ten, twentii, thiry, forty, five-ty." I put them away.

"The bigger ones are nickels, five cents apiece."

I thanked her with my eyes. "…twentii-fife, thiry, forty, forty-fife." I looked at her for confirmation.

"What happened to 35?" she asked.

"I forgoot dahat."

"Okay, so remember it. Now count the bigger coins, the quarters."

I looked at her inquisitively.

"Twenty-five cents," she said. "They're a quarter of a dollar."

"Oh, yeah, that's right." Simple lost things were easily regained. "'A course. Tweny-fife, unh, fifty-sity, sevenny-five, eighty."

"Almost." She took the coins and counted them up slowly so I could see. "That's 75 and one dollar."

"Got it."

"Well, not exactly. Now count the copper pennies."

"Could I use a clal-culat-cher?"

"No, you can't use a calculator." She crossed her arms and looked at me like a skeptical genie. It seemed odd that I should know what a calculator was and not a quarter, but such are the quirks of brain damage.

Money clearly wasn't my forte anymore, but there was no way in hell that I was going to continue to rely on my mother and my friends to cook meals for me. Kari taught me confidence by being my backup in the grocery store and in the kitchen. She gave me back the kingdom of cooking while I reclaimed the whole wide world of my imagination.

***

I now had few opinions on the subjects that I had once mastered: Craters of the Moon National Monument, the Owyhee Canyonlands management, the 9 million acres of proposed Idaho Wilderness on the maps I had helped draw, Wilderness Study Areas on Bureau of Land Management lands that I had collaborated with Katie Fite in mapping. The federal laws that I knew by heart, the subjects in which I had 20 years of learning, were only acronyms now: ESA, FLPMA, CWA, NEPA, NFMA. What did they mean?

I could relearn the facts and acronyms easily, but it wasn't the office I missed. It was the challenge of my work. I loved my environmental work because winning was always a fight in Idaho, and it required creativity. I put my heart into the drills Lynae and Kari gave me to make the environmental work more relevant, and by October they were bearing fruit.

Once, when I was feeling particularly discouraged, I decided to go visit Merritt in Washington D.C. I didn't feel capable of talking much on the phone with her, so it seemed like a good time to get my courage up to fly. Finding my way through the airport, taking off, the altitude, the motion, the landing--the complexity of it all threatened me in a way that is now hard to understand. But imagine yourself as a caveman walking into the 21st century. This was how I felt when I rode from Pocatello to Boise or flew to Washington D.C., when pieces of everything that I knew seemed so brand new.

Merritt met me at the airport in Baltimore, and we drove to the Capitol Mall. We lay on the grass in front of the Washington Monument, stretching into the sky above us, and watched lightning bugs flicker like shimmering stars in a vast darkness.

"What would you say if I said I wanted to move west?" Merritt bit her lower lip.

I was shocked. Would she really want to move closer to me? That would be wonderful. I was confident that I could regain my skills, but the process might be messy. How could I show her I loved her and wanted her? "How 'bout Boise?"

"I've got a job that would let me do my work by e-mail."

"Great!"

She gave me a tight, quizzical smile. "Would you like that?"

"A course."

"Well, I can't move for about six months."

"Six weeks?"

She smiled. "I'm not sure where I'll live. Maybe Reno or Denver."

"Yeah. How 'bout Ketc-hum?"

"We'll see."

The sounds of humanity were far away as we watched the fireflies blinking. Remarkably, Merritt loved me with all my brand-new deficits and old impetuous ways. She was now my best friend, delighting me with her insightful comments and repartee that sometimes cut to the bone. She was harsh but fair when I brooded over the effects of my stroke, charming at the most unexpected moments, winsome when she was sleepy and unprotected. Those times when she was vulnerable, with her cat purring near her heart, were the times I loved her most intensely.

After the passage of three months, Merritt rented a car in D.C., packed it with furniture, books, and everything else that fit, and invited me to come along with her. We discussed several places where she could live, and she decided on a nice apartment in Hyde Park in Boise. Her employer paid for her office a couple of blocks away. And would I help her move in? Of course! This was my luck: The man who never thought he'd find love, had been given this chance. She gave me what I couldn't find without her.

It was great to have her in Boise; we could go to movies and concerts, go on hikes and bike rides, and get to know one another more intimately. Now that she was in Boise, Merritt said that she wanted a dog since I had a real backyard for her to run in. It would be my obligation to house the dog. "Sure," I said "We should get a dog." We discussed this over a cup of coffee at my place.

"Let's just go to the pound and see what we can find," Merritt said with puppy–like enthusiasm.

"Ok," I said mindlessly. It was a sleepy Saturday and the temperature was already nearly a hundred degrees at high noon. I was barely awake but the coffee was finished, and she led me by the hand to my car. We got on the freeway and drove to the dog pound, which, much to my annoyance, was open.

Merritt coaxed me out of the driver's seat and into the blasting, brutal heat. All I wanted was cool air and another cup of coffee.

"Oh, come on, Mike, quit being a stick in the mud!"

"I, uhh, don't know if I wan a big old slob-blobbery dog."
I was pleased about how that came out.

"Let's just take a look."

"Oh-kay." I sighed.

We walked into the concrete floored, canine-smelling pound, and entering into this world put a positive jolt of caffeine in my cup. Dogs barked and people smiled as we wound deeper into this dogland. We filled out paperwork, and were paired with dogs that Merritt and I picked. Merritt pulled a leash out of her handbag--which seemed like a setup to me-- and clipped it to a little male beagle. We walked him out back to a grassy spot behind the pound, which was groomed for dogs to walk with their potential masters. "Sit," Merritt said. He sat down and we backed away from him. He wouldn't come to the most enthusiastic calls. We thought he must have been badly beaten by someone. He wasn't for us. When we took him back to his cage, his kennel mate jumped all over him while he cowered.

"Let's check out that jumpy one," I said, so we took the knee-high, brown and white, saddle- shoe looking little dog out into the yard. She seemed very glad to get out of that restrictive cage and was wild, running all over the lawn--which was to Merritt's annoyance and my pleasure. She was clearly not well-trained but she came when we called her for the third or fourth time, after tangling with a dog that another couple was controlling more effectively. I had to admire her spirit.

"Mike, I don't think she would work out. She's a Brittany, and I had one of those when I was growing up. They're impossible! Besides, she doesn't look like she's house-trained."

"We've come over a few odher ob-stacles," I said. We tried out three more spiritless dogs before leaving the crazy kennel, and we agreed that we would talk things over before returning to pick one. It wasn't going to be an easy decision, Merritt insisted.

Oh, but it was, I was thinking as we drove through the doldrums of the day. After I dropped Merritt at her house, I drove back to the dog pound and got the Brittany. There would be hell to pay, but after all, the dog would be living at my house. It was a spontaneous decision, and I hoped against hope that Merritt would be pleased.

"That dog is a disaster," Merritt said when I brought the Brittany over to her apartment. She petted the dog. "As long as you're willing to deal with her messes it might be all right. But you'll have to get her a dog license, get her shots, get her a collar, feed her, and care for her."

"Oh yeah, I guess I could do that." If I remembered.

"Mike, she is *your* dog." No, Merritt was not at all pleased. "Why don't we try her for a week?"

"Yeh. Unh huh."

In a week, the Brittany had been a devil's twister inside my house. She climbed on the dining table to see outside and badly scratched the walnut finish of a beautiful three-leaved table my mother had given to me. She tore into my New Yorker magazines, ripped the side off a lovely basket that was a gift from a woman I'd met before the stroke, chewed the covers off of a journal, and annihilated two books that I hadn't yet read. One morning there was a pile of shit and another puddle of puke for me to clean up when I awakened. Later, she tore into the upholstery of my formerly nice car—and I mean tore into it: the door frames, dashboard, and steering wheel had teeth marks and gouged material, as if the devil had ripped up the inside looking for hidden drugs.

Merritt said, "Your choice, Mike." But when the Brittany got out of the house and was captured by the dog catcher, it was Merritt who brought her home from the pound. She laughed when the dog climbed a tall box elder outside the kitchen window in search of a squirrel. Both of us laughed when the dog suddenly barked uncontrollably at a fire hydrant that she'd calmly walked by the day before. A moment later Merritt added, "Mike, I should also tell you that the people at the pound said she kills chickens."

"Thanks, Merritt. I'll keep that in mind."

We'd come up with a few names for the Brittany, but the one that stuck came from a meadow outside Fairfield as we traveled to Redfish Lake near Stanley. The field was brilliant with cobalt Camas flowers. We called the dog Camas and she ran like a hard prairie wind.

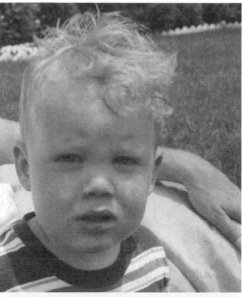

Right: Surly kid Mike.

Below: A promotional shot of dad pretending to be a tough cookie in L.A..

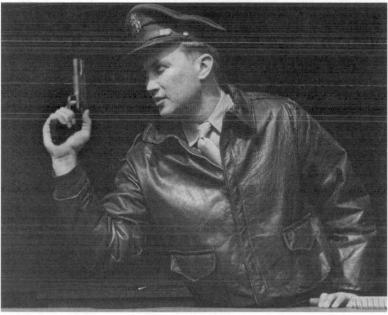

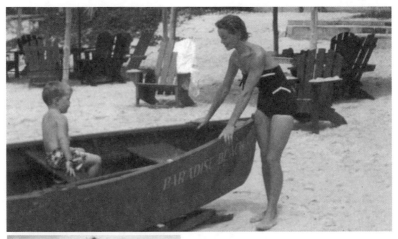

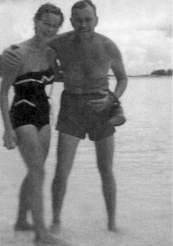

Above: Young mom and me at the beach.

Left: My mom and dad on the beach.

Below: Promotional shot of mom in Japan in the 1940's.

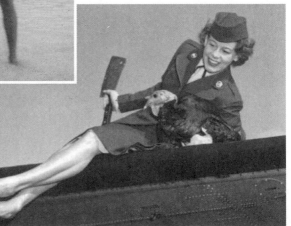

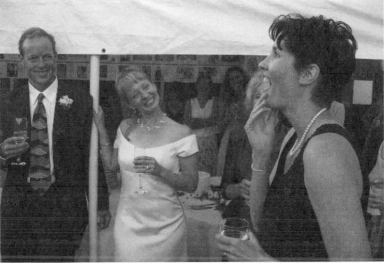

Mindy's inspiration; a fabulous tale of wicked times past.

photo by Diane Ronayne.

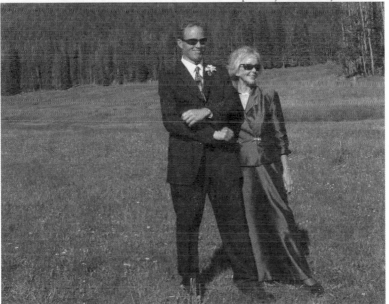

Mom and me at my marriage with Merritt.

photo by Diane Ronayne

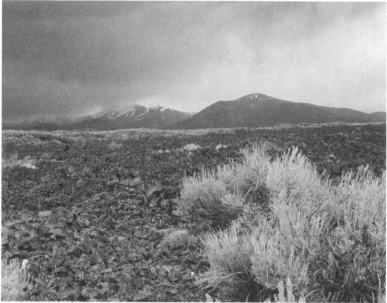

The coming storm on the day of my stroke.

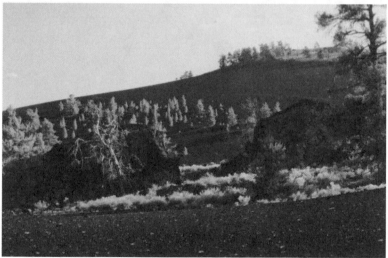

A cinder field and limber pines in the Craters of the Moon area.

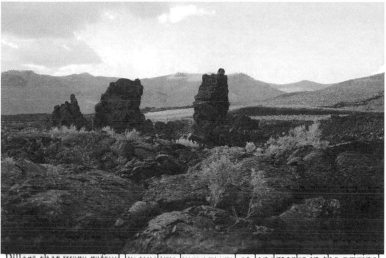

Pillars that were rafted by molten lava served as landmarks in the original monument.

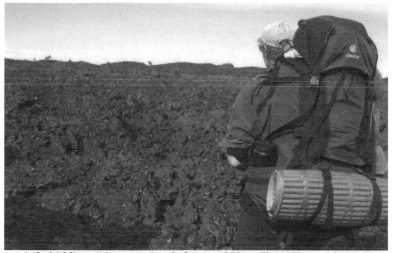

A forbidding sight as we headed toward Vermillion Chasm, through rugged A'a lava.

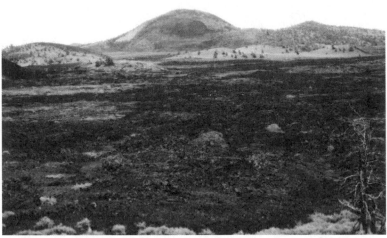

An overview of the wicked terrain that dominates Craters of the Moon.

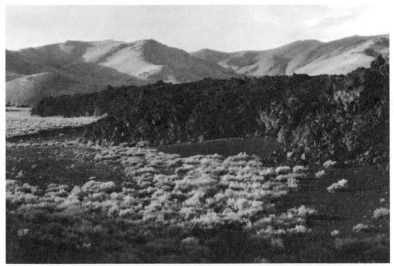

The end of the A'a flow of lava and the beginning of the
Pioneer mountains.

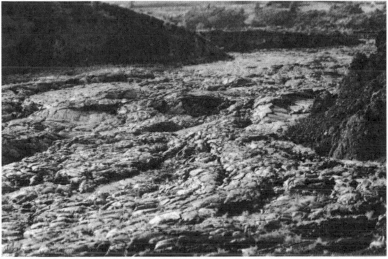

A frozen river of pahoehoe lava.

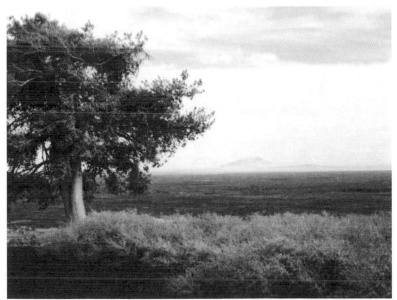

Pinion pine before the view of nearly invisible Big Southern Butte.

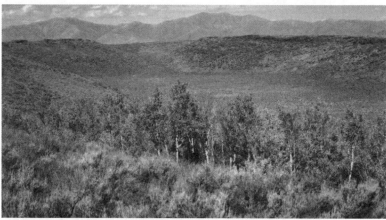

Aspens in Snowdrift Crater where Secretary Babbitt and a group of
ranchers met to discuss expanding the national monument.

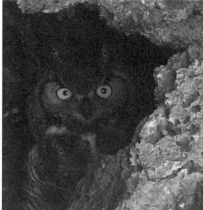

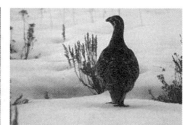

Above: Rare sage grouse are not
an uncommon a sight in winter.
Photo Courtesy of NPS.

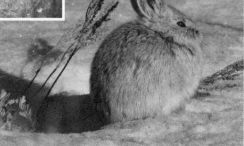

Above: A great owl
peaks out of a cave at
Craters of the Moon.
Photo courtesy of NPS.

Right: A threatened
pygmy rabbit at Craters
of the Moon.
Photo courtesy of NPS.

Healing My Soul

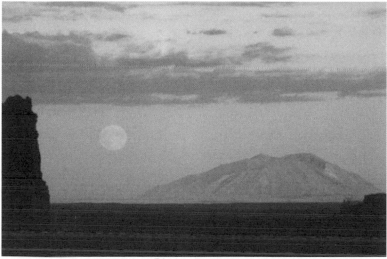

A place to contemplate - Big Southern Butte, the moon, ramparts, and miles and miles of the most desolate and beautiful lava country in Idaho.

Photo courtesy of NPS.

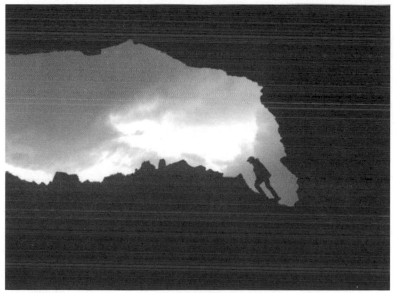

I climbed out of darkness and into light in the Craters of the Moon Wilderness.

On the Dark Side of the Moon

Chapter Four

Healing the Land

In late November 2000, I heard on the news that President Clinton signed the proclamation expanding Craters of the Moon National Monument to 737,000 acres. It was a done deal. Just like that, the President had protected nearly three quarters of a million acres with a stroke of his pen. Clinton's proclamation stated, in part:

The kipukas provide a window on vegetative communities of the past that have been erased from most of the Snake River Plain.... As a result, the kipukas represent some of the last nearly pristine and undisturbed vegetation in the Snake River Plain, including 700-year-old juniper trees and relict stands of sagebrush that are essential habitat for sensitive sage grouse populations... The most recent eruptions at Craters of the Moon took place about 2,100 years ago and were likely witnessed by the Shoshone people, whose legend speaks of a serpent on a mountain who, angered by lightning, coiled around and squeezed the mountain until the rocks crumbled and melted, fire shot from the cracks, and liquid rock flowed from the fissures as the mountain exploded.

On the Dark Side of the Moon

The proclamation expanded the national monument by nearly 14 times its previous size. This 410,000 acres of the new land would be managed by the National Park Service on the Great Rift while Laidlaw Park and 400 kipukas within the Rift area would be managed by the Bureau of Land Management, along with "undisturbed vegetative ecological communities," which amounted to 327,700 acres. The national monument now had two different management directives: the Park Service mandate to protect and interpret land and wildlife for the public benefit, and the BLM's to ensure "multiple use" for all. The two services would have to work together to manage the monument.

I was happy about the proclamation, naturally, but I had played little role in getting the last-minute work done. I couldn't help feeling discouraged and depressed about doing so little for such long stretches of the summer and autumn except waiting for the grass to grow so that I could cut it again. On the positive side, though, I could push the lawnmower, and I was alive. What I didn't know is that much more work would need to be done to heal the Craters of the Moon landscape, and that this was just another step in a longer-term process.

Early in 1924, Limbert went to Washington, D.C., with the draft of his National Geographic article in hand in order to advocate in Congress for protection of Craters of the Moon. "No more fitting tribute to the volcanic forces which built the great Snake River Valley could be paid than to make this remarkable region into a national park or monument," Limbert argued. Congressman Addison Smith of Idaho took up the cause and enlisted Interior Secretary Hubert Work to help persuade President Coolidge to help the protection effort.

Craters of the Moon National Monument was established by President Calvin Coolidge in May 1924, shortly after Limbert's visit and the appearance of his article. In his proclamation designating the 54,400 acre monument, Coolidge called it "an area which contains a remarkable fissure eruption together with its associated volcanic cones, craters, rifts, lava flows, caves, and natural bridges which are of unusual scientific value and general interest," and noted that it "has a weird and scenic landscape peculiar to itself." The creation of the national monument was a fine but partial victory for the broader Great Rift.

Forty-six years later, in 1970, the Craters of the Moon National Wilderness of 43,243 acres was designated by President Nixon under the Wilderness Act of 1964. This was another partial victory for this vast lava country. In 1989, democratic Congressman Richard Stallings from Idaho, proposed expanding Craters of the Moon from the original 54,440-acre national monument to a national park of nearly 400,000 acres, with an additional national park preserve of roughly 120,000 acres. Congressman Stallings hoped that a national park would give Idaho a tourist draw, the panache that the nearby towns of Burley, Pocatello, and Blackfoot areas lacked.

I had been working for the Idaho Conservation League (ICL) for a few years as its public lands director when Stallings announced his proposal. The ICL had already been working to protect Craters, particularly the grassland kipukas within the lava flows and the Wilderness Study Areas (WSAs) on Bureau of Land Management property. The 490,571 acres of WSAs were identified by law as protected until Congress either designated them as fully protected wilderness or specifically released them from that consideration. The WSAs were protected unless Congress identified them as developable, but, in truth, the WSAs in Craters were covered in lava and there was no demand for their use. It is precisely the demand for use that drives the need to protect land by limiting competing uses on it. Whether the issue is wilderness hiking, mountain biking, mining, live-stock grazing, or other uses, heated conflicts are inevitable.

The extravagant grasslands in Laidlaw Park kipuka emerged as a focus of major conflict between native values and grazing of livestock for private profit. If Laidlaw Park wasn't included in the BLM national conservation area, any designation would solve little for the region. If it was included, ranchers would complain bitterly because their income might decline. This wild and handsome place hardly knew a human footprint. However, it showed the significant impacts of cows and sheep, along with the predator killing techniques employed by ranchers. I was amazed that so few people in Ketchum, the glamour spot in Idaho, had ever been to Craters, even though it was less than 50 miles away. With a hundred or so vocal, informed people, we might have succeeded in designating the kipuka and Craters of the Moon as a national park or a national conservation area, but most locals seemed to have little interest in Craters. No one, myself included, thought to invite the public, who were the users and owners of this public land, out to Craters and divine if they had strong opinions about how it should be managed.

Local ranchers, on the other hand, had every incentive to involve themselves in this concern, as it directly affected their interests. They were an influential force in the communities around Laidlaw Park, in the towns of Carey, Arco, Picabo, Minidoka, and Rupert. Ranching was their bread and butter. No cows out in the kipuka meant no money; lots of cows, lots of money. The Marlboro Man, the fictional and commercial hero of TV and magazine fame, still had the sympathies of the public, so there was really no need for ranchers to organize. It was that simple, and after Stallings ran unsuccessfully for the

Healing the Land

Senate in 1992, his proposal faded with no one to carry the banner.

I went to Laidlaw Park for the first time in the early 1990s as a representative of ICL. It was an obligatory "show-me" trip with a BLM team and a group of ranchers whose main objective was to get a water well drilled for livestock--and to get the BLM to pay for it, naturally. The BLM representatives included the resource area manager, his assistant, a research assistant, and a quiet but credible botanist. The ranchers, John Peavey, Bud Purdy, and Pete Cennarussa, had a great deal of clout among them. Peavey was a well-respected state senator, Cenarussa had been the assessor of the state of Idaho for 30 years, and Purdy knew every pebble of this landscape, every state official of note, and most of the famous people who came to Sun Valley, a fact that gave him a good deal of influence. I stood in the middle of Laidlaw Park and nervously spoke my piece. It didn't go well at all; the only people listening were the BLM officials.

However, the ranchers eventually did come to support a study for a proposed Area of Critical Environmental Concern (ACEC) in the northern side of the park--the main area ICL was concerned with--as a tradeoff for an environmental assessment of the economic and environmental costs of drilling the well. Of course, it would be paid for by the BLM, but that was no problem for any of us—it was Uncle Sam's money. The study was needed, and I was in no position to oppose it. It was a victory for the environment to a degree that none of us fully recognized at the time. And to their credit, each of the ranchers loved the land and said that they wanted it maintained in general good health, but it was Cennarussa, a long-time sheep rancher, who acknowledged the specific goodness of protecting the landscape.

On the Dark Side of the Moon

It proved economically infeasible to put a well way out in the north park because the water was far too deep and therefore too expensive to bring to the surface. The ACEC study showed that the grassland was in good enough condition to be brought back to its native condition. This was in contrast to the rest of the Snake River Plain, with such dominant species as cheatgrass and halogeton, which was impaired beyond restoration by constant, heavy livestock grazing. The study also determined that a variety of native plant species were still present in the area in a quantity that surprised me. Such small victories added up to a killer of a study, conducted by BLM botanist Steve Popovich, and it laid out all of the right reasons for establishing an ACEC and protecting Laidlaw Park. This small northern quarter of the kipuka had remained relatively unscathed by the severe overgrazing that had turned the vast Snake River Plain into a cheatgrass hell. Many millions of acres of the open range had been destroyed, but this one last enclave remained as much of the Intermountain West once had been.

If a 20th-century cowboy had told ranchers about the damage cattle would do to the West in a hundred years, no one would have believed him. He might have told of the effects of the tall grasses disappearing, of waterholes drying up, the elimination of grizzly bear and wolves and eagles, the fouling of rivers, and trapping, shooting, and laying out poison to kill whatever might find it in the Western landscape. Who could plan such damage to the land and still make a living at it, knowing as he walked out into the sagebrush what the future held? Robert Limbert would have laughed at this mythical cowboy, yet his photographs documented that decline. The incremental change could barely be observed in a decade, but it ate up the land's productivity in the span of a human life. And now it was coming to the point of ecological disaster.

Healing the Land

Cheatgrass, that short-growing, nonnative grass in the south and central portions of Laidlaw Park, was highly inflammable and would burn rapidly and completely in any significant fire, scalding the land and reducing the ability of the land to recover. Livestock pools that had been bulldozed over were now full of feces and urine from cows; their filth killed native fairy shrimp in the pools and brought disease to native wildlife. Cows de voured nutritious native plants, leaving the ground bare and vulnerable to other invasive plants that wildlife wouldn't eat. The grasses that journal writers in the 1800s had chronicled as abundant, and at times "up to the knees of a horseback rider" were scarcely present by the end of the 20th century over much of Southern Idaho. This desert country had been pummeled by domestic livestock and was in dire need of whatever protection it could get.

In 1994, at the beginning of President Clinton's first term, former Idaho governor John Evans wrote a letter to Interior Secretary Bruce Babbitt proposing the expansion of Craters of the Moon as a national monument. It read:

Stretching for nearly 60 miles across the Snake River Plain, two large lava fields are considered the best example in the world of basaltic volcanism that can be appreciated in a short time and that is in an accessible location. The Great Rift is the deepest known open volcanic rift on earth and the longest in the continental U.S. . . . The designation of these lands has the potential to help the small communities around the area without infringing on traditional uses of grazing and hunting. There is strong local support for this designation and support among the Idaho delegation.

Craters was just the sort of place Secretary Babbitt wanted to hear about and he heard about it in a report from the reputable University of Idaho. It appealed to his professional training as a geologist and his longstanding environmental concerns. In 1999, at Craters, Babbitt embraced Governor Evans' idea and the bones of the expansion proposal advocated by Congressman Stallings years earlier. He gave a speech about protecting diverse landforms through the creative use of different land management mandates and jurisdictions, giving both the BLM and the NPS a common goal to protect large landscapes. This template was already succeeding in New Mexico's El Malpais National Monument and National Conservation Area, which had been designated by President Reagan in 1987. El Malpais was like Craters, an area of lava managed by the National Park Service, and its national conservation area included BLM lands that were used for grazing and hunting. This was a perfect model for the Craters of the Moon area, as Molly McUsic had recognized when Katie Fite and I met with her in her office in Washington D.C.

Babbitt's authority came from the Antiquities Act of 1906, a federal law that allowed the President to declare deserving land a national monument by proclamation, just as President Coolidge had previously done for Craters in 1924. That power hadn't been in Stallings' hands, because creating a national monument wasn't his goal. He wanted a national park, and that couldn't be accomplished by presidential proclamation. But adding land to the existing monument was a way to sidestep the legislative process. The curmudgeonly, quixotic Republican-controlled Congress in power in 1999 would never have approved the designation of Craters as a national park. It was a bit unilateral to use a law that had been passed in 1906, but Babbitt figured it would do the job. The grazing and mining interests had their share of unfair laws on their side, so this was a fair trade for the public.

In his proclamation, President Clinton would have to identify what was of historic or scientific value at Craters of the Moon and designate what the Antiquities Act labeled "the smallest area compatible with the proper care and management of the objects to be protected." Fortunately, there were plenty of big objects to be protected: lava flows and kipukas, rare plant communities, unique animals, curious volcanic formations, and the Craters of the Moon Wilderness Area. In addition, the Shoshone Indians had used the area since prehistoric times, and tribal members' testimony about their lore, legends, and love of the land would give the proclamation quotable spice.

Idaho Senator Larry Craig publicly criticized Babbitt for not going through the public process and failing to abide by the National Environmental Policy Act (NEPA) by not preparing an environmental impact statement. It was an ironic statement from Craig, who had never shown much interest in following NEPA guidelines, but that's politics. Clearly, Babbitt hadn't had to perform an environmental impact statement because the Antiquities Act superseded such standards. Craig sought to defeat the proclamation by delaying the approval process indefinitely, but he was thwarted by the Antiquities Act. Rep. Mike Simpson issued a press release that said, "The debate should be driven by the community and the best way to ensure lasting support is to allow the community to develop a proposal, on its own, and bring it to Congress. We simply don't need the Antiquities Act anymore." The congressmen from Idaho were furious that Babbitt had the power of the Antiquities Act and would ignore their partisan interests, but the Republicans didn't have the necessary majority in Congress to eliminate it. Rep. Simpson also

failed to realize that Republican President Reagan had done exactly what President Clinton was proposing.

The first time Babbitt came to Craters of the Moon in April
of 2000, he flew by helicopter to the southern Wapi flow. Here
he saw Crystal Ice Caves, a place where icicles had grown drip-
by-drip for millennia that had nearly been lost through BLM
and concessionaire poor management. The massive stalactites
and stalagmites in this cave had melted as a result of warm air
flowing through a new vent that concession owners had cut
into the rock as a way to let customers see the beauty. Mel
Kuntz, a U.S. Geological Survey geologist and long-time student
of Craters of the Moon's lava briefed Babbitt about the Caves
and nearby King's Bowl, a dramatic 500-foot sink in the lava.
After a couple of hours, they flew along the Arco-Minidoka
dirt road and back north across the Great Rift to the National
Park Visitors Center, where Babbitt held an impromptu news
conference describing what he had seen.

The second time he came, I was struggling with my stroke
in Pocatello. The story came to me through personal conversations, press clippings, and my knowledge of the place. Babbitt came armed with a map, and after meeting with ranchers
in Arco, they drove the 50 dusty miles to Snowdrift Crater in
the vast Laidlaw Park kipuka. He had planned to meet with
people who made their living off the land, those whom would
be most affected by the designation. It was a brilliant plan for
him to see the Craters of the Moon country, talk with ranchers
about it, and attempt to resolve the differences. At the rim of
Snowdrift Crater, the group stopped and piled out of their cars
to gaze down a 150 foot drop to the flat bottom of Snowdrift
Crater. They looked at a handsome copse of aspens standing
where no trees should, surrounded by miles of brown and olive
desert shrubs. There was cool shade here. It was a landscape

that normally varied only in small distinctions of color, but now, with the aspen leaves newly green and sagebrush and bitter-brush flowering and encouraging sneezes, the contrasts were stark and spectacular—brown and green against white clouds floating and a deep blue sky with the sagebrush fragrance of the Intermountain West wafting through all of it.

Everyone followed a path between the cliffs down into the aspen grove. A dozen men and women crowded Babbitt as he disembarked from the government-issued van, and they walked side-by-side down a steep brushy hill to a flat spacious place where they could sit and talk with Babbitt's collaborators.

Rocky Barker, a reporter for the *Idaho Statesman*, tagged along like paparazzi in a helicopter following Secretary Babbitt's collective on the road. Later he told me, "One of the magic moments of my career was when I watched Babbitt lay out the maps in Snowdrift Crater with the ranchers, Purdy, Peavey, Cenarussa and Rochelle Oxarango and asked the group: "What should we do?""

The question held in silence, so he answered it himself in that Jimmy Stewart way that Babbitt spoke. "Well, here's what I think," he said. Babbitt ran his finger in circles on the BLM map indicating Laidlaw Park and the Wapi Flow. His gestures captured the whole area of the Great Rift, including all of its kipukas, the Wapi Flow, and the Crystal Ice Cave to the south. Babbitt's proposal also included Laidlaw Park, the 50,000-acre halo of sagebrush-steppe grassland within the Great Rift that was, at that time, being grazed by livestock. He pointed to the map and asked again, "What do you have in mind?""

Barker, a reporter with an opinion about nearly everything, was eager to give me his when I interviewed him more than a year after the meeting happened in Laidlaw Park. He's a genial guy who has watched environmentalists expand their power over the years. I'd known Rocky for a decade and argued with him about a variety of points—we still do--and we never came to agree about the proper role of environmentalists. But then, we never discussed the roles of journalists either, who often left out the drama among people, which were the guts of any decision. "This is just how federal land management should be done," Barker said of Babbit's work. "Neither the off-road vehicles nor the enviro interests were there to veto it. Babbitt had the federal power and the Antiquities Act, and that put President Clinton's power in Babbitt's hands. They decided to create the monument, and that's what happened."

Barker grinned and his eyes sparkled as he recalled the scene. "Part of the magic of the moment was that even people who had turned against wilderness were fighting for the monument," he said. Barker added that Babbitt's staff compiled all the information that he received from the Idaho Conservation League, The Wilderness Society, the federal agencies, and Governor Evans to justify the monument.

Even people like Arco rancher Bob Waddoups, who had opposed protection for the wilderness, would now support Craters because of Babbitt's assurances that the area would not be opened to mining, that the federal land could not be sold, motorized vehicles would be limited to existing roads, and hunting and predator control would continue to be allowed. And, of course, livestock grazing would be allowed in areas where it was already practiced. That was exactly what the ranchers wanted, and it amazed me that all of this happened without much clear influence of environmentalists. I had to admit Rocky was probably right about the role of the environmentalists—we're better at forcing the issues than at resolving them. We argue and spit and never seem pleased. However, we got much of what we had wanted at Craters of the Moon by fram-

Healing the Land

ing the conflicts and pushing the issue. And so did the ranchers. The compromise, therefore, seemed a good one.

Indeed, the points had already been decided upon by the time the parties came to a public meeting in Rupert, Idaho a few weeks later. This consensus included management of the Great Rift by the National Park Service, and Laidlaw Park and all of the kipukas within the lava flow by the BLM. The agencies with differing mandates--the Park Service as the preserver of places for scientific inquiry and public enjoyment, and the BLM for multiple use and conservation—would have to work together to manage the new monument cooperatively.

The ranchers who helped create this consensus were mostly content with what Babbitt offered because they trusted him. What Barker said was just what happened: Babbitt heard the arguments on all sides and planned to propose the Great Rift as an enormous monument: it was going to favor the economics of rural Idahoans and ranchers. What was going to change in management on the ground? Not much.

President Clinton issued the Craters expansion proclamation using the Antiquities Act in much the same way that President Carter had in 1980, when Carter and his interior secretary, former Idaho Governor Cecil Andrus, expanded Alaska's Arctic National Wildlife Refuge by several million acres in the dying hours of Carter's presidency, when nothing could be done to reverse the decision. After the contentious election of 2000, however, George W. Bush came into power, and the policy on Craters of the Moon took another turn.

In 2002, Congressman Mike Simpson wrote legislation that summarily changed much of the new Craters of the Moon from a national monument to a legislatively protected national preserve, a designation that allowed hunting on and around the lava. Hunting is entirely prohibited in national parks and monuments but is allowed in a preserve or a wilderness. It is also allowed within BLM and NPS wilderness study areas. Simpson argued that his constituents in Idaho favored hunting and quoted from Clinton's proclamation, "Nothing herein shall be deemed to enlarge or diminish the jurisdiction of the State of Idaho with respect to fish and wildlife management." Now we all had to live with these words, which were the result of the compromise Babbitt had crafted out in Laidlaw Park's Snowdrift Crater. It was a promise given and unfulfilled by the federal government, until Simpson wrote the national preserve legislation.

The new national preserve legislation also gave the area specific statutory protection, through an act of Congress. Full congressional approval was far stronger than a presidential proclamation, which, though legally enforceable, could be changed or revoked by a subsequent president at his discretion. An act of Congress would not be so simple to change.

In practice, granting hunting privileges amounted to virtually nothing, as few would seek to cross rugged expanses of lava to hunt antelope, deer, and other wildlife that weren't living there in significant numbers. Regardless, it would surely be a slow and painful way to hunt, and at least the national preserve language was concrete. The National Park Service supported it and only a few people opposed the legislation. It was signed into law by President Bush in August of 2002. The Park Service now managed 410,000 acres of a national preserve, and the BLM managed about 327,700 acres as the Craters of the Moon National Monument; both now allowed hunting, with the exception of the original National Monument.

Today, the BLM has responsibility for the larger kipukas, like Laidlaw Park, Padelford Flat, and Little Park, and the agency continues to allow livestock to graze in the preserve. The proclamation language, which forbids mining claims on the entire monument, was retained in designating the preserve, but then again, there has never been mining in this area. Multiple use, which is one of the defining mandates of the BLM, means that every land use has to be considered, from grazing livestock to allowing off-road vehicles, to hunting, to bike rallies. The National Park Service policy, by comparison, is simple and transparent: no cows, no hunting, no poisoning of predators, no mining, no logging, and no motorcycles or off-road vehicles would ever be allowed in the untracked backcountry of a National Park. That was compromised by negotiated provisions in the national preserve designation, and the proclamation consensus points were preserved by Congress.

This philosophical difference between the BLM and the National Park Service harkens back to environmentalist John Muir's arguments, for preservation of the land versus conservationist Gifford Pinchot's desire to utilize resources such as timber, minerals, cattle, and a multitude of other uses. This controversy still largely defines the use of public lands to this day, with few exceptions.

However, one area that transcends the division is the provision under the Federal Land Policy and Management Act (FLPMA) for wilderness study areas, or WSAs, on lands managed by the Interior Department. In areas more than 5,000 acres that are not roaded, the land must be preserved as it is until Congress determines its suitability as wilderness under the Wilderness Act. The FLPMA applies to both the BLM and the NPS, which are Interior Department agencies. Wilderness Study Areas comprise 471,200 acres, or 64 percent, of the Craters monument, encompassing both BLM and NPS land. The FLPMA has protected millions of acres of the American deserts and temporarily preserved them as they may have looked 200 years ago, before settlement. The WSAs stand unchanged within the monument and continue being protected—although not permanently--unless they are identified by Congress as deserving wilderness designation. But that seems a distinction without a difference; this land remains wild.

So was Babbitt's original compromise or the national preserve legislation a defeat for conservationists? I think not. The monument and preserve legislation has done more to retain the status quo than to enhance firm protection of the area, but the grand landscape at Craters now has more certain information associated with it, which encourages ranchers and environmentalists to maintain the lands' unique natural values, along with the economic value of maintaining livestock grazing. Federal law, defining the preserve's values, will assure that each is protected.

Conservationists aim to protect many values of the land, its animals and plants for example, and in the process we may recognize that some things, like grazing, need not be so damaging to the land as it had been in the past. I have been changed by the hard path I've travelled and so have ranchers. This was exactly the lesson for me of having a stroke: getting well will take time, each step will bring painful progress, and I cannot always get the things that I wanted. This is my healing path toward recovery, and learning is not a bad compromise in life.

Four years after my stroke, Gov. Babbitt told me, as we drove together along a highway in southern Idaho: "I think that in Craters, what we foresaw happening was...not much." He chuckled. "We wanted to get out ahead of the problems and make the designations before the conflicts could arise. The only thing we foresaw that would be of immediate concern was a more careful attention to Laidlaw Park and administration of grazing and control of off-road vehicles." He paused for a moment, looked at me, and then added, "The proof will be in the management plan that they (the BLM and Park Service) are starting work on and that was mandated by the monument proclamation. The BLM has been very slow about getting started on those monument plans and that is where you judge their intentions: when we see whether they are serious about effective regulations and whether they put resources into enforcement. I don't think we know yet. They have just been slow starting."

The management plan for Craters of the Moon National Monument and Preserve has been long in coming, but it was a healing process. The plan was finalized in 2007, but it would be an iterative process, responding to the needs of the public within the confines of the law. The plan identified management actions that returned the land —slowly— to what it might have once been, and the details of incremental occurrences over many years have made it possible to recover. We are all evolving.

On the Dark Side of the Moon

Chapter Five

Recovering the Present

A few months after my mental and physical therapy ended in 2001, I came across the work of Dr. Antonio Damasio, a leading neurologist, writer, and professor of the brain. He would be speaking that autumn in Sun Valley, just west of Craters of the Moon, at the Sun Valley Writers Conference, and I decided that I should be there to learn a thing or two about the brain. I could even write about his lecture to pay for the trip and might visit Craters afterwards because it was close by. Sun Valley was one of my old stomping grounds, so I could just camp out there and visit friends. But first and foremost, I wanted to ask Damasio a few questions.

Damasio was talking to a colleague of his when I arrived at the big tent where the conference was in progress. I had contacted him prior to coming to Sun Valley, and he agreed to chat with me. When he finished his conversation, I rushed to introduce myself and we sat down at a nearby table in the sun.

"Ok, I've got about 15 minutes," he said. Damasio has European good looks. He is Portuguese, about five foot seven with a stunning streak of gray swept back in his otherwise obsidian hair. Under the blazing sun, I started with the big question: "What is consciousness? What makes it critical to human endeavors?" I say the "big question" because I felt I had lost a major part of my consciousness when I had the stroke and that pain endured, even after my rehabilitation had ended.

Graciously and directly, he replied, "Consciousness is a way of knowing and feeling your existence in our surroundings. It is one of the great creations of our brain. It really is a way of endowing our own mind, our own imagination. It's really something beautiful--the sense of our own body, our own organism being modified by our action, by our perception." As he spoke, he gestured with his hands and arms, then stopped to think and made his fingers into a tent of air. "In other words, constructed at the floor of consciousness is something called "the self." The self is an image we have of our own body changing when I, for example, talk to you, when I touch something, or when I hear something." He looked at me to see if I was following.

"Ok, so, consciousness is our ability to know," he continued concisely. "It is something that is constructed in the brain, and it is entirely connected with the body. If we didn't have a body, of course, we would go out of existence. We would never know the end. But our consciousness is not something that is given, that side is a revelation. There is an internal connection. That's the beauty of it." And, I thought, the deep mystery of it as well. Consciousness is "the unified mental pattern that brings together the object and the self," as Damasio wrote in *The Feeling of What Happens.* "Nearly the whole brain is engaged in the conscious state." But I had found that recovery came in pieces and at odd times. I asked him, if there was hope for people who'd had brain damage, whether from accidents, disease, or other failures, to recover their losses.

"I think that there are a tremendous number of possibilities. First of all, the results of the stoke." He paused. "What types of symptoms did you have?"

"I had a left-side stroke," I said.

Recovering the Present

"Left side of the body?"

"Left side of the brain. I think what it did was damage the Broca's and maybe the Wernicke's areas." Damage to Broca's area in the brain prevents a person from producing speech properly and any speaking tends to be slurred or slow. Damage to Wernike's area of the brain results in the person being unable to understand the speech of others; often they may speak clearly but fail to make any sense, confusing the meaning of words. I had a combination of each effect, both of which eventually diminished significantly.

"Did you have paralysis?"

"I had paralysis for a few weeks, and I've tried to get control of that and pretty much have."

"How old are you now?"

"Forty-five."

"So. First of all, what you get when you have a stroke totally depends on which parts of the brain are involved. Anything could be involved, from memory to emotions, language, the motor system, perceptions of every kind. The possibility of recovery is very much related to the size and scope of the stroke. That's one thing, but it's also related to age. It's related to intelligence and to education. The people who do better with their strokes are young people and people who are intelligent and highly aware of themselves and have the willpower to respond to that difficulty."

It was hot there in the sun, and drops of sweat formed on his forehead. I figured I had time for one more question: "What are the possibilities for recovery from a brain accident?"

"It is easier to treat strokes now than it was 20 or 50 years ago," he said. "There are many ways in which this has become easier as more medications have been developed. And there is also something which is very important: It's the thought that, because the brain is very plastic, because the brain can be re-hearsed, there is practically no end to recovery. You can always get slightly different systems of the brain, systems that were not affected, gradually to take over some of the functions that were lost, by doing the functions not in precisely the same way but in new ways. For example, what you lost in the damage to Broca's area can be recovered if the damage is limited. And you have recovered, obviously, and that's why you are doing perfectly well. If you hadn't told me that you had had a stroke, I wouldn't know without examining you first. There are many areas that can be compensated, but there are some that can't."

"Why is that?"

"Look at it this way. Imagine that you have a system of pumps, and they bring water from here to a variety of places, and you have all sorts of relay systems in the pumps. If you damage one of the peripheral pumps close to a certain area, that's going to cause very little trouble. But if you damage something that is very close to the main trunk of supply, you're going to create a heck of a problem. And it's going to be a lot of time before you can bypass that system."

Damasio answered all my questions in the 15 minutes we had together, and it all boiled down to this: Consciousness is a process, an endless rehearsal. It is a way of knowing and a gift to think. I would have to endlessly rehearse every valuable skill that I wanted to master. I wanted a miracle, of course. I wanted to recover fully. I wanted alchemy; I longed for dull lead to become gold, and that simply wouldn't be.

I floated in ether, and finding enlightenment would be a longer process than I ever imagined. Although I'd made a lot of progress, I wasn't satisfied with my life because I couldn't do what I had chosen to do a few years ago: to protect part of the natural world, make a fair living, and to find love. I thought about Craters of the Moon which was roughly 39 air miles to the southeast. I should have been there now. I missed it like a friend, but there were other things I had to accomplish first—like knowing more about myself. That place would wait and I would go there in time.

In the meantime, I chose to go to a workshop entitled "Using Media Effectively," in Boulder, Colorado, to regain some of the professional skills I'd lost. It was offered by The Wilderness Society, my former employer in the 80s, and was like classes I'd attended half a dozen times before to get tuned up on the latest theories of communications.

The workshop was held in a university classroom with cinderblock walls on a cool summer morning. The sun was out, and it warmed me through a window in a hallway as I watched people come and go with spiral notebooks. I wasn't sure I wanted to go into the conference room. I lingered until I got cold standing in a breeze, and then I slipped inside.

It had been difficult enough learning media skills the first time, and now my stroke had upset everything. I was back to the starting line. I had forgotten key concepts and didn't speak well enough to be on camera. Why should I want to be on TV or radio? To be an advocate for wilderness and to make the case for wild places, I supposed, but I now felt hopelessly insecure. I couldn't remember enough for more than one sound bite, though sometimes one was all it took. I had to trim my sound bites to make each word count, each phrase quotable.

I went to the workshop with my good friend Doug Schnitzspahn, who had found me on the lava. He was learning about the press, reporters, tape recorders, and cameras, as once I had, and he wanted to go to a mock press conference to gain experience. I wanted to recapture the most basic skills. We moved together in our different ways.

On the Dark Side of the Moon

A woman was arranging chairs in a large circle when Doug came in. We sat down as the chairs filled. There was a sense of excitement in the room, the thrill of learning something important. Soon, it was jammed with people. The workshop leader, Tia Hinson, waited for us to quiet, and then began talking intimately, almost in a whisper.

"This workshop is going to be about love, and passion, and the real feelings that the press never reports," she said, flicking her smooth black hair as if shooing a fly.

Real feelings? As opposed to what? False feelings? I felt scared. I wasn't the jaded pro I had been a few years ago when feelings were easy to convey. This would be a whole new experience for me. I considered bolting, getting the hell out of the building, but people were standing in the doorway, blocking the easy way out so I sat and listened.

Tia introduced a man and turned the forum over to him. "Getting good press," he said, "is about returning to the place where I first felt a real feeling." He gazed into a corner of the room as if remembering something from the distant past. He threw a piece of plain white paper down in the center of the circle of people. "This is the place you will speak." He stood on it. "This is the place where I begin to feel," he said, and held a dramatic silence. Victor had a thin nose, a bony face, and a voice slicker than butter on a hot summer day. "I remember feeling alone. I closed my eyes when I was hanging in a tree about twenty feet off the ground. I was afraid to fall."

Hanging in a tree. Nice image. Where did this guy come from, Ore-ree-gun?

Victor continued. "I was in a dream where there was no one around, and I felt danger. I was alone and vulnerable. I felt cold and weak. I didn't cry, but I remember that's the place where I started to remember it all." He closed his eyes.

I wished him the best of luck in keeping his story together, but I thought again about why I was here. I sat tight.

"It felt genuine. Not false. I stood out from the other people and said something they wouldn't agree with. I didn't want to fall from the tree, and I wanted to make them believe me. It was a tragedy in the making. Then the bulldozers came, clearing the wild forest so that builders could start pouring concrete." He opened his eyes to punctuate his point. "I found so many things there, things like slugs, birds, ferns, a coral snake, lizards--the things that could not be replaced. So many people just thought the building houses thing was inevitable." His eyes bulged. "How very real that felt for me that day!" He swirled the colorful braided bracelets on his arm. "That's the point. I had to get to feel like I was genuine. There was a risk to take. And right then" --his fists clenched and rose before his face-- "the cameras rolled."

Nice story, but a bit simple. I decided to get out of this classroom with the ebbing tide, while there was a lull in the presentation, and I stood up to leave. Before the cameras rolled.

"You," he said suddenly looking at me. "Could you read me this poem, 'Witness?' It's by W. S. Merwin."

Oh, shit, I was caught. "I uh, don, unh read so goot out-lod."

"That doesn't matter. Just take a chance."

"I uh differ." I wanted out of that room, fast. Suddenly I was terrified.

"Just a little two-liner." He held the silence again, waiting for me to choose.

"Uh...Ok." He handed me the piece of paper. The poem was short, like he said, two lines. I read it first to myself and then out loud. "'I wand to tel-yu whad de foresds wer like, I will have to spek in a for-gotton lan-lan-guage.'" I butchered those beautiful lines. Then I stood there naked among strangers and friends, ashamed of my voice, cadence, and pronunciation, ashamed of myself. I hid behind a secret that no one knew. It wasn't me. It was simply what I had become.

"Thank you," he said.

I sat down, shaking, and didn't dare say another word. I was stuck to the seat by the glue of embarrassment. Well, this was a workshop, after all, and I sure was getting some concise practice.

Victor asked for another volunteer to read a longer poem. This one, by Robert Frost, was about a man who takes a walk through an area of dilapidated homes that were almost indistinguishable from age. This man gets lost beyond finding himself, but he finds himself in another way. A woman read the poem perfectly, and silence fell again.

Victor beckoned another person to rise, and she told a story that was simply too fabulous to believe--she was the heroine of some kind of knight-errant tale. As I thought this over, another woman stood up and took three deep breaths, clearly breaths of anxiety and import. They conveyed: "I've got something I've wanted to tell you for practically a century, and here it comes. I've been waiting to tell you, now listen." I did. The whole room full of people did. She was genuine, no doubt about that.

She fidgeted and fought back tears. Being part voyeur, I looked for the tears, the sweat in her armpits as she raised her arms over her head, the shaking as she spoke. She suddenly smelled like a gymnasium. She tossed back her long red hair, and stared out at the quiet, hot room full of silent people. Her look was of a cold, hard fear held in check as she bit her lips. She took another long breath and stepped onto the piece of

paper that was the speaking place. I believed her wholeheart-
edly before I even knew what this spellbinder was going to say.
There was a sense of electricity in her actions, impulsiveness.
She looked stricken and compelling, beautiful in a helpless sort
of way, thin and fragile. No way was I going to leave this room
now.

Finally she spoke. "I threw a piece of trash out the window
of a car once. My aunt sat next to my mom and me, and she
said that maybe it wasn't acceptable to throw trash out on the
road. I mean, I hadn't really thought of that, and I suddenly
felt humiliated." She looked at Tia. "You know how many
times I had thrown trash out of the car? You know, my mom
and dad did it and so did I. But my aunt was right." At this
she wiped her eyes, and took a big sniff, and sat down. All of
us looked at her helplessly. Where was the story? This was why
she worked to protect the land? Because she felt so bad about
a piece of trash once upon a time? But why the passion? Why
the emotion. Why was this such an issue for her?

Tia rushed over and hugged her and the woman laughed in
embarrassment. She had run out of steam, her anxiety spent.

In the uncomfortable silence, a dark haired man blurted out
that he once had a memorable dream. "No, I don't mean that I
was Martin Luther King, I mean it was real, I can't remember
exactly. I was walking on a stack of cut, peeled, and piled logs
out in the wilderness." He had a beard and stroked it, calming
his fear with this habitual gesture. Everyone in the room was
on edge.

Tia asked him to stand up. Oddly, he wouldn't stand on the
piece of paper to speak. He pretty much danced around it.
"These logs seemed like they were centuries stacked one on top
of the other with all the branches cut off. I felt terribly sad as
I walked on top of the highest one. I felt so damned angry! I

was pissed off that the timber company cut so many logs and just left them. They just left them to rot!" He raised his arms in alarm. "And I sat down on the logs and thought that the Potlatch Company cut and left them for so many years. They were just cutting more and more and leaving them to rot. That's what made me fight the timber company, the anger that I felt for Potlatch."

Abruptly the man sat down. A couple of other people told about their defining moments, but none said anything related to the media. Then the workshop was over, but no one wanted to leave this sweaty, smelly, crowded room. There had been nothing about the media in any of this; it was all about motivation and belief. Well, maybe that was what it was all about; believing passionately in something, believing passionately that we have a story to tell that is worthy to report. But why didn't I tell my story of having the stroke? I couldn't say. Because it was tough and embarrassing?

Victor stood once again and waited until people saw and focused on him. "Speaking gives us consciousness," he began. My mind rolled over that statement: "Speaking gives us consciousness." No, that's not true. Not at all. I disagree! I was snagged on those words: consciousness…speaking…consciousness…. I didn't hear another thing he said, or notice when he finished. People clapped and slowly drifted away. A few stood around talking in low voices.

I sat looking blank, thinking about consciousness: being aware of thoughts, feelings, actions, impressions, memories; an endless rehearsal, giving a gift to myself, knowingness. None of them involved speaking. Did they? When I didn't speak after the stroke, did that mean that I didn't have consciousness? Absolutely not! I stared at the window opposite me, and the trees beyond it with sun in their arms. I was angry. What Victor had said was backwards—exactly backwards. Wasn't it?

A woman I had befriended many years ago approached me. "Hey, Mike, you ok?" She was a kind and gentle woman, but firm in her beliefs, and she saw me looking out the window blankly. I wanted to hug her and say a warm hello.

My eyes burned as I looked at her. "No. No, I'm not. "How are you?" I burst into tears and sobbed for a long time on her shoulder. She was as surprised as I was: to be a virtual stranger crying and holding onto her. I claimed her shoulder as a place to cry--a violation, but she didn't flinch. Strong women have always amazed me at their capacity to understand sorrow.

Tears spoke for me. She hugged me, and her own tears rolled down her cheeks like tiny silvery pearls. "I've got to go," I said emphatically. I held her eyes for a moment. "I am alive." She nodded and wiped the tears from her cheek and smiled at me.

"I'm glad," she said. I walked away, knocking into a chair with a clatter that drew attention to me.

I went outside into fresh air. I was a writer, and now I could barely form words, much less form meanings, and write them in coherent lines. The words counted, and their loss hurt. Maybe that was what Victor meant. I had been to the point of having my consciousness fail, speaking gibberish, my mind in free fall. Consciousness and thought were in suspension on the lava: I didn't know what I knew. In the hospital where I was deposited, I only knew what I didn't know. My paltry language, and feeble mind, and not knowing what I once knew had brought me to grief. Knowing that I was not able to reach at knowledge taunted and tortured me. Victor had put his finger on it. No, he was wrong. *Speaking does not give us consciousness.*

On the Dark Side of the Moon

*To speak, first I must think. To think, I must want to know. To know,
first I must be aware. But where was this awareness, this consciousness,
found? Was it in confidence, self-respect, fortitude, or creating my own
damned good luck?*

I want to tell what the forests were like
I will have to speak in a forgotten language.

But I didn't know the words of that language.

I ran down the street in Boulder so I wouldn't see anyone I
knew. I ran in fear and found an outdoor shopping mall to
wander in and wonder. What kind of place was this? I felt uncomfortable, angry with all the people sleepwalking from store
to store, restaurant to bar, going somewhere they planned to
be. I controlled my anger by looking at my reflection in a pool
of water. Why was I angry? I watched the artificial stream flow
down the mall into this pool and disappear.

Soothe me, clear water, calm me.

*Was anyone awake? Was anyone full of the blood of life and con-
nected to this piece of earth? I looked around; everyone was lost in thought,
in the future, in the past, everywhere and anywhere. But not here. Where
was here? I saw dozens of people; I saw their sweaters, skateboards, skis,
and shoes coming out of stores. They looked happy and pretty. I felt my
losses burning like a hole cut into my head with an acetylene torch; I was
neither happy nor pretty.*

*This time was all that people had, all of them, every single one of us,
and look how we were spending it. I wanted to holler something profound.
I ran to grab a man with a black beard and stared at him. I wanted to
scream but I just stared into his face. He was bewildered and pushed me
away with a derogatory remark. I was a weirdo.*

Where was I? I'd lost myself and the stars to navigate by.
I felt myself spinning out of my mind. I sat beside the phony
stream, put my head in my hands, and cried tears of self-pity.

Recovering the Present

After a while I walked on through the mall and found a black man playing congas beside that little phony waterfall. He wore earplug headphones and muttered an odd tune and smiled at the day. I closed my eyes and sat close to him, listening to the rhythm: tak, tak, atak, pakutat, boom, paku, mat-atak, tat, tat, tak, tak, tak, atak, ratutak, rat-a-tat, thrum, thrum, thum... It was insistent, pounding, and I sank into its cadence and enchantment. He played louder. Surely this was a jungle sound. I thought of Craters of the Moon and the music of the land. I thought of the Shoshone. Inside me, I felt black trunks, and palm fronds above--the Te leaves of Hawaii, water falling off a cliff into a river, vines hanging in air. That was his tune. Or mine. I imagined all the people passing by me surviving in the bush together, alert, vibrant, and aware of the wild world around them. This mall was a place to gather food. Everyone was alive and playing a tune of their own. It was slippery magic, sparks-and-phosphoric magic in the brain: worlds stolen from thinnest cerebral tissue. I slipped into a trance.

My mind faded away and I walked in darkness with a friend from my youth in Sacramento. I told him there are only two ways I can go: to the darkness of wilderness in the tangled brush beside the river where I grew up, or towards the streetlights glaring on a shiny black street that holds the glow of footprints for a moment as people walk along.

"Dave, I'd like to go this way." I point to tangled brush.

He laughs and spoke like Groucho Marx. "Ok, Mike, I'll see you later at your apartment." He fiddled with an invisible cigar. "I'm not headed your way; it's much too muddy and wet. For me. I'll get us a pizza. If you don't show up, I'll eat it." He tapped the cigar to shed an ash. "I'll eat it anyway, my friend"

On the Dark Side of the Moon

I head for the woods and vines and trees beside the American River. In dim moonlight a great horned owl flies by and tells me, "I will take you where you need to go." I follow, stumbling through brush, wading in ankle-deep mud. The rich river odors of life and decay--of anise and fig and overripe grapes--mingle with the reek of spawned-out salmon. The owl lands on the branch of an oak tree, and I sit before it and watch until the moon runs down the horizon and the sunrise reveals the shapes of morning. I am immune to the passing of time. The owl flies away and I am sitting beside the river, which is skirted with debris. Far beyond, light on mountain tops graze the Sierra Nevada. I try to see where the path I came by leads, but there is nothing at all to see, no trace of my passage. Just nothing, until I see that this is a path that I chose to walk long ago. It is no path at all. I'm simply here--alone.

My steps have led me here today, and this time is mine to live, with the losses, the gains, and all the beauty. There is nothing to follow, no trails, no footprints. There is no path. One day I ran a half-marathon to Robie Creek in Boise, a healthy man with no stroke risk factors, and the next I was on my back dying on the lava. There was no "why" about it--no one to give me an answer, no one to blame, no one to cure me. It just happened that way. And now I'm here at the beginning again, not recovering my past—that was lived, past, and gone—but trying to reclaim the present.

***

The man nodded at me and continued playing the congas. I left to wander the restaurants and shops of Boulder like a shell-shocked soldier, watching people but no longer judging them. I sat motionless on another sidewalk bench, thinking about what I had become, until a man shook me by the shoulder.

"Mike, Mike, there you are!" Doug laughed when I opened my eyes. "I've been looking for you. Let me buy you some lunch." I stared blankly at him. "Are you ok?" he said.

"Uhm, yes, yes I'm, unh, fine." I nodded and wiped the tears and smiled. I had learned nothing concrete today, but I recieved a glimpse of myself and the loneliness of humanity. When I thought of all the other people, with their insecurities and infirmities, their attempts to communicate with words spoken, unspoken, and written, their fear of mortality, the undeserved diseases that would surely kill them--well, what did I have that was so different or so crushingly bad?

I had forgotten to care about my fellow human beings and their foibles and this entire insane and outrageous world. I had forgotten self-confidence, compassion, and companionship, and I had come to loathe myself. I had forgotten the plights of others in feeling so sorry for myself. I had forgotten that every person is walking a unique path. In my anger, I had forgotten what mattered in my life—the stroke had erased even that. It was my love of people and of nature. I sat beside a tree and watched this oblivion die. Compassion was the language I'd forgotten a long, long time ago. It is a wordless language.

This world was just fine with all the odd and infirm people in it, and I would start all over again, learning from the beginning. *No, I can't do that. I can't erase the past. I can't fail to remember having a stroke or the effects of it—the good and bad. But, this time I'll live my future with a little soul and lot more joy.* There was still plenty of work ahead, but I had a friend who would buy me lunch, and that seemed like a good place to start recovering.

***

A few months after returning from Boulder, I proposed to Merritt in a Thai restaurant in downtown Boise. The setting was colorful, decorated with scarlet silks and bright paintings. She said yes, she wanted to marry me! The diners beside us clapped as we toasted one another. I felt excellent, brisk, and strong. Merritt looked radiant, natural, and happy.

After deliberating and planning for what felt like half a century, we got married in a stunning meadow below the Boulder Mountains surrounded by 150 friends. It was one of those perfect days offered by the mountains around Ketchum. Everything went well and our merry friends danced and drank to joyous excess. We drank champagne, ate chocolate mousse cake, and endured unmerciful teasing by the wedding party. We danced a swing and spun like tops, as blissful lovers should, but in a wink the evening turned sharp and cold. Our families and all the partygoers left, and we waved them farewell as we took off on our honeymoon.

We drove up and beyond Galena Pass and stayed at a lodge in the foothills of the White Cloud Mountains, looking west to the Sawtooths. To the southeast, Craters of the Moon laughed with us. It was Eden for a few days, and we reveled in it: horseback riding to a dinner spot in the woods, basking in hot springs, looking at the mountains that once had been my home, and hiking in flowery foothills. All that lacked was the soundtrack to "The Sound of Music," but the silence proved even better. We were in love like adolescents.

A few days later, I ran out of money. We had flown to Hawaii to continue our honeymoon, and at the airport in Lihue my credit card ran dry. I had expected it to last for the two-week trip, at least, but alas, I had gone on a bit of a spree. Merritt paid for the car rental, hotel, meals, and most everything else, to my shame and her astonishment. This was the price of my stroke, I rationalized. We stayed on a beach in Hanalei, Kauai, walking in tide pools and snorkeling beyond the surf in a world of oddly finned fish: sergeant majors, angelfish, and stingrays. We drove across the island finding string-of-pearl waterfalls and pineapple stands offering fresh, tangy, succulent fruit. We read books and drank fabulous smoothies of pineapple and mango. But I still had no money.

I had planned for us to hike the 22-mile round trip on the Kalalau Trail along the magnificent cliffs of the Na Pali coast. The path slithered high on the cliffs, with drops of a few hundred feet in places and 1,000 in others. We got the backpacking permit I'd sent for a month earlier and made sure that we had all the equipment we'd need—packs, hiking boots, water bottles, stove, pans. But I hadn't planned on Merritt's fear of high places. She had never told me about that.

We walked most of the way, picking and eating wild mangoes, guavas, and passion fruit along the route. We were cooled by the fresh breeze and mist from a 300-foot waterfall and felt pure. Just as we turned back, at the midpoint of our three-day hike, Merritt froze up. All of a sudden, she couldn't take another step. We still had a lot of ground to cover, and the trail hugged the cliffside in either direction. Only a slim path crept along the winding precipice, with 500-foot drops below. I was astonished. She stopped and planted herself as firmly as a hippopotamus.

"It's ok, Merritt." I looked reassuringly at her, although I had my doubts. "It's no problem."

Merritt shot me a searing look that shut me up. Before I knew what was happening, she slipped and let out a coyote's scream. She clutched at grasses and wouldn't get up.

"I'm falling!" she insisted.

I said, as calmly as I could manage, "Don't worry, you're not falling. You're just sliding a little." Oh boy, was that the wrong thing to say! I was caught up in the ecstasy of the scenery, the cliff, and the endless ocean. Her situation didn't seem particularly dire to me, but these were not the most comforting words I might have chosen. She *felt* as if she was falling.

"Help me up!"

"Give me your hand…."

One of the tourist helicopters that flew the Na Pali coast hourly, all day long was hovering right above us, and I imagined the muffled voice of the tour guide: "If you look out the right side of the helicopter, you will see a pair of honeymooners struggling with their relationship on the most precipitous cliff on the Pali. The Pali was a goddess who played with fire. And now, aren't you glad you took this trip instead of hiking along those wicked cliffs?" Turning like a Sky King pilot, the man and his tourist ship fell away like a stone and pummeled the air with a whop-whop-de-whop giant eggbeater sound.

"Help me!" Merritt screamed.

My hand shot to her and she grabbed it, slowly pulling herself up. We walked to a boulder where she could sit and regain her composure. Her confidence was shattered. She shook and inhaled deeply and looked out to the flawless turquoise ocean for several minutes. We got up and walked a few steps, and then she was in control. She said nothing as we hiked out the long Na Pali Coast to the end of the trail. I felt bad now as well as broke and I owed her whatever I could give. We sat in our--or her--rented apartment in uncomfortable silence and slowly warmed up to one another as we ate dinner with a bottle of too-expensive wine. It was only then that I remembered Merritt's fall as a child. She had been crushed by her horse when it spooked and fell back on her, and she'd spent years recovering from the accident.

"I nearly died," she said, breaking the silence.

"You nearly died," I agreed. "I'm really sorry." It was etched in her memory and there was no sense in my aggravating her. The truth lay in her perception of it.

Two days later, we flew back to Boise to live in my house beside the foothills. It was our home now, and Camas still climbed the tree out back in search of squirrels. My lack of a meaningful job and my money problems were our problems now as all the little obligations came pouring back. Merritt had a mercurial nature—she was full of love but angered irrationally. I wanted her to be consistent but I couldn't acquire her patience for a pile of gold doubloons. Sometimes we mixed like vinegar and baking soda, and at other times we hiked in bliss for a week, but it was always worth the risk to make our love work.

On the Dark Side of the Moon

Chapter Six

An Unbearable Beauty

I still had a lot more healing to do when our marriage began. I wasn't angry anymore, or not most of the time, but I was deeply sad, and I knew no one wanted to hear my carping. They'd heard it. I didn't want to project my sadness on Merritt, my mother, or my friends, but I didn't want to keep it all inside me, either. It hung over my mind like a black cloud just waiting to burst. I decided to take a journey back to the scene of my disaster, to confront it at its source and try to recover my joy in living.

Again, I read Robert Limbert's *National Geographic* article about his 1921 trip to Craters of the Moon. It was the sort of place, he wrote, where "one wants to feel free from human interference, to be able to gaze and feast their eyes on the scene spread out below without being molested... It is here that one feels little and insignificant, a fly on the wall of the world. The desire of conversation is lost and one is glad when he is at last free of the crater rims that tower overhead." Limbert's nickname was "Two Gun Bob," earned during a tenure with Buffalo Bill's Wild West Show, in which he would toss a silver dollar into the air and shoot a hole in its center, or so he bragged.

I wanted those towering crater rims, and that silence, and the powerful sense of awe to soothe my aching soul. Going back to Craters of the Moon with Limbert as my virtual guide, walking along the route of his journey, sounded like just the tonic I needed. It would be a solo trip out to the oddball ends of the national monument, ending in Laidlaw Park kipuka, the place where my epic had begun. I planned to search out many of the fantastic formations Limbert described and see whether they had changed over time. My trip would coincide with negotiations over the joint management of Craters in the wake of President Clinton's proclamation expanding the area of the national monument and Rep Simpson's bill for the preserve, so perhaps I could make a contribution to the final debate.

Limbert began his trip near the town of Minidoka and traveled north through the Great Rift lava flow toward Arco, near where the Craters of the Moon visitor center is today. He brought along an Airedale Terrier, and he wrote that in only a few days the dog had bloodied his feet on the razor-sharp lava and had to be carried for much of the two-week exploration. Limbert was a booster and showman who knew a creative name when he heard one. It was largely through his article that the name Craters of the Moon stuck to this lava landscape. In 1923, geologist Harold Stearns explored Craters at the behest of the U.S. Geological Survey, and wrote that the landscape was similar to "the surface of the moon as seen through a telescope," an observation that surely influenced Limbert's rhetorical flourishes.

Among many striking features of the Craters landscape, the Blue Dragon Flow was a particular favorite of Limbert's. "It is the play of light at sunset across this lava that charms the spectator," he wrote of the Blue Dragon. "It becomes a twisted, wavy sea. In the moonlight its glazed surface has a silvery sheen. With changing conditions of light and air, it varies also even while one stands and watches. It is a place of color and silence." The Blue Dragon Flow, although named by an earlier explorer, was ideal for a promoter like Limbert. It sounded like it could be a moving beast, a monster who breathed magma in every fiery breath, its scales rippling with opalescent brilliance. This flow is unique to Idaho and shimmers because of the titanium that rose to the surface during ancient eruptions.

Vermillion Chasm, the Bridge of Tears, Echo Butte, Yellow Jacket Water Hole, Trench Mortar Flat—each of them a geologic curiosity within Craters of the Moon--were named in the course of Limbert's hikes. Only an inventive mind like Limbert's could sway President Coolidge and win his support for this landscape. Limbert wrote that it was destined some day to attract tourists from all over America. But they never came. Tourists never flocked to this parched land in the hordes he'd expected, but it wasn't for his failure to tell wild stories of stunning caves, surprising arches out in the desert, fabulous cinder cones and hidden water holes, diverse lava flows and enisled kipukas, abundant wildlife, and striking, colorful miniature flowers.

Limbert was a jack of all trades: an outfitter, an ardent sportsman, and a writer of short stories and poetry. His photos of the Owyhee Canyonlands documented grasslands that have since been despoiled beyond recognition by livestock grazing. He photographed the abundant grasses that grew along Idaho's Snake River and the justly famed Shoshone Falls, the waterfall immortalized in a painting by Thomas Moran. One of Limbert's photos shows him and his Indian brand motorcycle beside fabulous petroglyphs. Today, those same petroglyphs have been all but obliterated by graffiti and are barely discernible and Limbert's work provides irrefutable evidence of the impact of careless use on the landscapes he cherished.

On the Dark Side of the Moon

He died young, at age 48, while returning by train from a speaking tour of the East in 1933. According to biographical material in his collected papers at Boise State University, the cause was a brain hemorrhage. When I read that, it stunned me. Someone about my age, who was an avid hiker, apparently in good health, had a stroke that mysteriously killed him. What else might Limbert have done? Where else would he have lived? I read his writings, studied his maps and photos, read his short stories and his obituary, and I almost died a similar death. He seemed a kindred spirit to me, and a little like my father, who would have loved to know a character like Robert Limbert.

In May 2002, I set out on my journey to retrace Limbert's route. I didn't bring an Airedale, as he had. I brought Camas, my little Brittany, who was small, mischievous, and raring to go. I drove from Boise out to the Park Service's loop road, the one my mother and I had followed a few months after my stroke.

Driving along, I saw signs about the places we had visited together, including the Devil's Orchard, named by a minister who said it was as close to hell as you could get without actually going there. I smiled wryly at this now, thinking that I had been there in hell. There were no devils and no brimstone out here, nothing but big blocks of basalt and a scene worthy of a desperado shootout. There was no one here to shoot at, though, only memories, but I was here to confront my past to save my present. The only hell was in my mind, and I drove on, leaving the Devil's Orchard to a more innocent breed of tourists.

Over the last year, my friends had gone on with their jobs and their lives as if nothing had changed. Of course, nothing had, except for my life. I was still having trouble with memory and language and feared having another stroke. For a while, I'd given up running, something I'd done for more than 25 years for the sheer joy of feeling strong and alive and being out in nature. "Free as a bird in a banyon tree; I'm the original happy me," was the way Hawaiian songwriter Kui Lee had sung the feeling when he was 21, about two years before his death from leukemia. It seemed to me that Kui Lee's was a noble life, a brave death. I'd lost my sense of freedom and happiness and had fallen out of step with my peers. That's why I'd come here: to regain my happiness. For joy. For strength. For peace of mind. To build confidence. To laugh again. To re-define who I was. To think, just a little, about *nothing,* and to listen to the silence.

At the end of the road, I parked and pulled my backpack out of the back seat of my car. I'd packed a three-gallon water jug, a sleeping bag, food for Camas and me for three days, maps, and a compass. Camas leapt out of the car like the very embodiment of happiness and the pleasure of living. I laughed at her joyful bounce..

Craters of the Moon was peaceful. Its views were expansive and silent, the landscape undisturbed by humanity, the flowers and vegetation surreal in the slanting light. Shades of black and gray absorbed poisonous thoughts like charcoal. Gray-green vegetation grew on raven lava. The blue sky glowed and the stark, unembarrassed land stretched out a long, long way, across the broad plain. I couldn't imagine feeling forlorn here; it just didn't make sense to me in this world of oddest beauty, this vast blackened wildness. I did not feel lonely here; I felt good in the silence, with nothing to explain to anyone.

The afternoon remained calm. Camas curled into a ball beside me as I made a late lunch—two hunks of homemade bread with millet and sunflower seeds, smeared with lots of peanut butter. Camas was illegal in the eyes of the park rangers, or so the signs told me. It pleased me that Camas, the dog whose name was a flower, was an outlaw here. That disreputatable dog had eaten the insides of my car for the second time. My auto insurance had covered the first episode of Camas' assault on the upholstery, but I had been warned that they wouldn't pay for a second outbreak of Angry Dog Syndrome. I planned to put Camas in her crate every time we drove together, but I figured she'd quit the chewing, just as she'd quit most of her other bad behavior. She never stopped being angry at the world outside the car and never stopped chewing the inside, but after a year of owning her I could handle that--with a wince and a large dose of forced forgiveness. She was a scofflaw at Craters, and I let her be.

We walked on. The trails faded to nothing. We two were wispy spirits sneaking our way through this world. I found myself walking again in the volcanic Hawaii of my childhood, with Mauna Kea, Mauna Loa, and the fields of lava on the Big Island. I went back to my core, to the edge of the lava field where my father and I had walked, my father before he had his stroke. He was healthy and vital, the man who sailed between the Hawaiian islands in any weather. My mind sailed across time and place as I walked. Ray Medberry on the sailboat was a happy man. Marj found her happiness without him over the years and both found peace. Those thoughts satisfied me.

Camas and I walked in silence. Charred skeletons of sagebrush announced that a brush fire had burned through this landscape some time ago. At first glance, it looked as if it might have happened only yesterday, but the circles deeply inscribed on a sandy hill by new, tall grasses told me the fire was much older than yesterday. I was now out beyond the middle of nothingness, and that suited me just fine as I walked along Limbert's path in my father's lava, pondering my stroke. I wondered if Limbert had been exaggerating about his Airedale's bleeding feet as Camas floated over the sharp lava. But then again,

Camas was as light on her feet as a ballet dancer and was much more nimble than an Airedale.

The breeze blew gently through sagebrush, carrying the plant's pungent bouquet. Lava divided the landscape into, black and tan broken dashes. The sunset lit a smattering of limber pines in a drainage between grassy hills, with a backdrop of rawhide peaks in the Pioneer Mountains. Onyx clouds cut the sky into layers but left a single line of intense blue. Little bluebell flowers shivered in the wind like chilled kids and reflected the piece of sky. The whole scene pleased me unbelievably. I wanted nothing to change. I wanted to keep this moment and nothing else--nothing but the shadows of mountains, the burned sagebrush, the limber pines that had escaped fire, the blocks of lava standing before me, and the Brownian motion of the flowers. I wanted to stay right here, seeing all of this scene, feeling its pureness. In the silence of the wilderness I needed apologize to no one about my inabilities. I felt the independence of this place, and I began to feel whole again: arms, legs, back, brain, and a soul that had fallen to pieces were reknitting. The body and mind were working again out here in this desolation. Ask me about reality in this black and blue, cinder-covered landscape and I will tell you it is right before you: open your eyes to light, color, the contour of the land, to the Blue Dragon flow, and look beyond yourself into its dark subtlety.

How could I explain this to anyone, this incomparable feeling of gain and loss? And what of the unexpected gains? I never would have lived to love this powerful but seemingly dead land without taking a look around. I wouldn't have fought to walk or to speak without setting out on a path. I never would have seen the glowing magic in leaves and light, never would have known how much value life may hold without opening my

mind to the undefined. Never would have felt the void of losing every thing of value in life, and never would have won it
back inch-by-inch without the desire to love life's mysteries. All
I needed to do was to look and open my mind to its unlikely
magnificence. I petted Camas, who was frightened by the howl-
ing, hollow wind.

A few weeks before, a friend of mine had died unexpectedly at age 44. His name was Lee Mercer. He had been on his
way to lead a hike in the Jarbidge Wilderness Area, just over the
Idaho border in Nevada. He stepped out of the car, looked at
the distance, and dropped dead from a massive heart attack. A
doctor who was on the trip treated him on the spot, but he was
decidedly dead.

Just like that, death comes to our door. Airplane crashes,
car wrecks, cardiac arrest--you name it. Lee was a bearded,
growling bear of a man who told stories of the grizzly bears
he had met in the intimatcy of his wilderness. He never made
a lot of money, but he didn't need much to be happy; Lee was
honest and hardworking and knew volumes about wildness and
bears. Just before he died he had found a woman whom he
loved and who loved him. It seemed to me that he had as good
a life as anyone I've known; it was true to his heart.

Camas and I walked out past a trio of odd-looking, blown-
out craters, Broken Top, Big Cinder Butte, and Half Cone. We
went on to Trench Mortar Flat, past Coyote Butte, Crescent
Butte, and finally to Echo Crater, where we camped for the
night. I read Limbert's words in a copy of his National Geographic article which I'd brought with me. Camas and I lay
down in a pebbly place and I slept a deep, quiet sleep under the
stars. At daybreak, the sky was overcast and calm. A flock of
geese flew east, according to my compass. But the compass
needle deflected a little because lava contains metal and is mag-

netic. When I sat up, the needle swung south. That was the direction geese flew at this time of year, I thought. No, north. Hell, I wasn't really sure, and I was still easily confused about these concepts in the wake of my stroke. The closer the compass was to the ground, the more the needle deflected and read untrue. It was an unreliable tool in the lava fields, although generally true to the magnetic soul in the earth, a point that had to be taken into account. And when you knew its soul, you could figure out its declination. I had been counting on the compass to guide me to Limbert's caves, and I'd marked them on a map that had few contour lines and no reference points, because the landscape was mostly flat—as flat as a lava flow can be. Pure lava provides few clues, so I would have to navigate from now on by half assed hunches and outright guesses with this wildly erratic tool in my wildly erratic mind. But at least I knew where the sun rose and set.

Quietness surrounded me again in the morning. For someone who didn't talk much these days, I was perfectly happy to listen. The dry air seemed to suck up sounds, the sky to absorb whispers. Suddenly, Camas raised her head. A woodpecker pounded on a distant pine for a moment, and when the sound stopped, it left a solitary feeling. Camas ran to find the source, but she ran the wrong way. I laughed and offered her my compass.

Snags of stiff limber pine looked haunted in the pitch black lava. I kept thinking that something would break out, some decisive noise, a clash of cymbals, lightning bolts, or a falling tree, but nothing did. I heard no more birds once the geese passed, no more woodpeckers, no water trickling, no chattering of leaves. Never was a silver-tongued preacher so profoundly eloquent as that silence. Camas looked around, alert, but silence remained.

On the Dark Side of the Moon

The feeling of silence soothed my worries like a good friend that morning in Craters of the Moon. The sky hung, overcast with wispy fox-tailed cirrus clouds beyond piles of low hanging cumulus. I lit my stove to make oatmeal and coffee as the clouds darkened. With luck, the clouds would bring no rain. In my backpack I had packed a little touch of joy: I made coffee with cream and brandy. Then we set out. Every ounce of water jiggled and gurgled and weighed on me.

Camas and I climbed a cinder cone called The Sentinel, which thrust above our 5,600-foot high camp. We climbed it to look around at the view and to test my endurance, up a steep trail with cinders under our feet sounding like a walk in Rice Krispies. Flowers were everywhere-- bluebells, little yellow and white flowers, larkspur, spring beauties, and purple pentstemon, but they were very small because of the altitude and dry climate. Wild bees flitted among the miniature flowers in their dance of survival. I thought of Merritt as I climbed. I wished she could see and feel this country. Sometime I would bring her here-- but I always told her that, and I coveted this silence. Still, she would like it.

From the top of The Sentinel, Camas and I took in the view. The view included The Watchman looking as if molten lava had lapped up like waves on its western side. That made sense, as I'd read in a Park Service brochure that lava had come at least twice in the last 50,000 years resulting in some very complicated geology. I looked around and saw the land as the hands of a compass: Big Southern Butte providing an enormous dark landmark amid the flatlands to the east, snowy peaks of the Pioneer Mountains to the west, North Laidlaw Butte on the southern side of the monument, and Idaho's tallest mountain, Borah Peak, on the approximate north. It was a magnificent wide-open view of the north end of the monument, clear and crisp in this vibrant spring.

We headed south to North Laidlaw Butte and Laidlaw Park. I had been hiking north from Laidlaw Park when I had my stroke and would pass that way again. Now we walked beside the Little Prairie Lava Flow in the shadow of The Watchman and The Sentinel, keeping to the grasslands and avoiding the rugged a'a lava wherever we could.

The lava flows in Craters are a fabulous and complex territory, dramatized on one of Kuntz's geologic maps in splendid colors: emerald, jade, and turquoise greens, outrageous oranges, blues, yellows, browns, pinks, and a regal purple, each color representing the age of the flows, ranging from 2,000 to 15,000 years old. Kuntz, the geologist who had authored or coauthored several studies of the Craters of the Moon geology over 30 years, had accompanied Babbitt in the Wapi Flow when Babbitt proposed the monument. He knew and loved this landscape, and I could see his love of the land in the geologic map of Craters of the Moon. I talked with him near the visitor's center at the monument in 2002 as he led a trip for students through the lava. I was surprised to find this man who described the lava like a friend who offered his theory on what had happened here only as one possibility. The colors in the map seemed oddly emotional for such a scientific tool, hinting at molten rock splashed in brilliant hues onto the paper. And yet the color key defined the movement of liquid rock over thousands of years in precise scientific terms. According to the map, Camas and I were walking over 15,000-year-old sky blue lava.

We came upon a narrow, rugged flow of a'a lava that the map displayed in lilac tones. A young flow from the Holocene epoch, it was the route that only a fool would take through the shrubby Prairie across to Laidlaw Park, mapped in a shade of gray. We walked on the lilac strip, an isthmus of a'a and I was surprised that Limbert had also found it almost 80 years ago, though without maps. He also found many caves, the Blue Dragon lava, discovered an oddball arch, and plotted all of them. The caves were my ultimate goal, and I told myself that Camas and I would walk until we found them on this day.

Fire from the sagebrush burn I'd seen earlier had slithered through this grassland and stopped abruptly at the edge of lava. Camas and I hiked over the lava through thick, tall sagebrush that grew like nothing I had ever seen before. It was brambly and nearly impassable, with some antelope bitterbrush, tall grasses, and small forbs growing between the olive-colored clumps. I stopped to consider this remarkable expanse of brush, which was exactly what sage country should be, but wasn't at least anywhere that I had seen. Everywhere sagebrush grew in the upper Snake River drainage, perhaps 10 million acres, there was no such thing as dense, tall sagebrush. That plant community had been crushed and eaten by cows and sheep for more than a hundred relatively continuous years. The Little Prairie was the first view of real sagebrush country I'd had. It was a view right out of Zane Grey's cowboy novel *Riders of the Purple Sage,* and was stunning for the life it contained: lichens and mock orange, sage grouse and mourning doves, great horned owls, gopher snakes, squirrels, and pronghorn antelope, among other unexpected living things.

This Prairie held the kind of country that was here long before the Bureau of Land Management existed--country that gave cowboys reasons to wear chaps. I began to understand just what the coming of settlers had done to the wild country and the wild animals that belonged here--to the bison, wolves, grizzly bears, and sage grouse. There was a tangible absence of beings that no longer existed in this Prairie, like a lost American tribe. I felt the void.

"In wildness is the preservation of the world." This much-quoted statement from Henry David Thoreau had been on a poster in my room as I grew up. In it was a picture of an old man wearing a backpack climbing up a mountain. He seemed to be the soul of perseverance. But what did it mean? What world was he trying to preserve? Did it still exist? Was this world rhetorical and political? Did it have earth, air, water, wildlife, and human beings in it? What did it mean "to save the world" these days? Did it mean that bison and grizzly bears would soon return? "That which is broken is made anew," Lao Tsu wrote long ago. I could only believe that he was right, both for the land and for myself. His thought gave me hope.

I felt thankful for the National Park Service, which protected places like The Little Prairie from livestock grazing. I felt thankful for the designated shard of wilderness in the monument. This place, The Little Prairie, felt a world away from Laidlaw Park, at least if you wanted to see what this country once offered. Some say that there is more moisture in The Little Prairie than in Laidlaw Park and that accounts for the difference between the two, but a trip through both of them reveals that livestock grazing has made a far more indelible impact.

Neither the Park Service, the BLM, nor wilderness designation would bring the bison and wolves and grizzly bears back to Craters of the Moon. But I did see sage grouse in The Little Prairie— a far rarer sight in Laidlaw Park farther south. Their droppings lay like the flicked ashes of careless cigarette smokers out in The Little Prairie kipuka. They were thriving in the greater diversity of The Little Prairie. But grizzly bears and wolves could only live here for small parts of the year because of the scarcity of prey and the extremes of the climate. Still, it would be great to see a bear or a lone wolf out in The Little Prairie or in the kapukas of Craters. Bison, on the other hand, would only be in a vision.

We fought with brush along a tall ridge of a'a lava. The Little Prairie a'a Flow was where Camas and I chose to cross into another section of The Little Prairie where the brush gave out to bare, sharp, soilless lava. Here the a'a lava, even for 1,000 feet, offered painful walking, with no semblance of a trail. It was a rugged stretch of sharp, unbalanced rock.

Monolithic blocks of lava stood to three stories high in the middle of a'a flows. In this unearthly rockscape it took us about three-quarters of an hour to traverse the quarter mile to the other side of the lava flow. Camas jumped with enthusiasm as we approached the second half of The Little Prairie again. Her paws showed no signs of blood or tenderness. We spotted another lobe of the grassy, sagebrush covered prairie and took that route. I was eager to get to the caves. I picked out a tall pinion pine on the sagebrush flat across The Little Prairie, and we hiked the two miles to it. We were searching for the Bridge of Tears, Ampitheater Cave, and Moss Cave, all of which Limbert described in his *National Geographic* article, but when we got to the other side of the grassland we saw nothing distinctive. The landscape around us looked like a level plain of jumbled rock. After another hour of wandering, we saw a man-sized cairn that stood out on the lava from half a mile away. We headed there and saw another pile of rocks, then another, and another, leading us to the caves.

I spotted a foxhole descending into the ground. Taking my pack off, I climbed down into the hole and felt a cool wind blowing out of darkness. Camas shied away from the cave entrance, as if she had anticipated being invited in and had decided against it. My eyes adjusted to the darkness, and I saw a shaft of light from above that had encouraged a growth of moss on the cave's wall—Moss Cave! It was just as Limbert had described it more than 85 years ago. My flashlight was insufficient to see much, but the cave went in two directions, one for a short stretch ending in rock, the other for an indeterminate distance.

I couldn't believe I hadn't had the foresight to bring a decent flashlight. Ah, but for a memory. Still, the flashlight I had stuck in my pack was good enough for me to see the bumpy roof of the cave and water weeping off moss. Water, that scarce desert commodity, dripped steadily on wet dirt. Camas wouldn't come to my call, though she looked guilty about it. Seeing her spooked bewilderment was enough for me to take a hint that what I was doing was unsafe, so I climbed out again into the harsh sunlight of the desert.

We walked about 50 yards and found the Bridge of Tears, a lava arch that stood like a massive inchworm. I ducked under it and out on the other side, nearly running into a gnarled limber pine. I smiled as I remembered Limbert's account: "...we came upon a natural bridge of lava arching to a point where two cliffs of lava narrowed down. It had a 50-foot span, and from the floor to the roof of the arch was 15 or 18 feet. Its width was 75 feet. There was a pine tree growing under the east entrance. One of the party bumped his head on the roof near the edge, so we laughingly called this the Bridge of Tears."

From there we traveled east and found the cave Limbert called the Amphitheater. I climbed down a steep narrow chute that opened into a wide room with two levels. Again Camas hung back, spooked, as if devils were rising in the dust before her. She circled the hole, barking madly, as I descended into the blackness. It was as alien to her as the fireplug in Boise had been; she had jumped back at the sight of it on the street near our house, and barked incessantly while Merritt and I laughed at her. But this was a more serious concern for her, watching as I disappeared into a hole in the ground.

I explored as far in to the lower level of the Amphitheater as my flashlight would allow. I didn't want to climb around the upper level for fear of falling and getting hurt in the moody fragility of this forgotten cave. Shadows of bats swarmed in the darkness above my head, and I felt a distinct need to leave the confinement of this underground capsule, as I have never managed to get rid of my instinctive fear of the erratic flight of bats in near darkness. I couldn't see the roof now as my beam of light dimmed. Daylight called! There were no stalactites, only the residue of white calcium from water drips. I could feel its roughness on my hands and knees as I crawled quickly to get out.

Limbert had found more magic than I in this cave:

It is an almost perfect model of a miniature theater, with a circular, sloping auditorium, a miniature bridge of lava for the stage, an orchestra pit, backdrop, and domed ceiling. It is lighted by a six-inch hole in the roof....

Climbing down, we found ourselves on the east side of a room some 40 feet wide and 60 feet long, with a domed ceiling 20 feet high. As we sat on the north side, we beheld to the south a perfect stage.... It was almost an exact model of a modern theater. To the right of the stage a large rock jutted up; imagination might call it one of the wings...

We walked and crawled between a quarter and a half-mile.... Finally, the passage closed down until the roof was only 1 ½ to 3 feet high...and Martin and I crawled on about 200 yards, until we came to a place we christened Fat Man's Misery...

The roof throughout was covered with stalactites and the floor with jagged drippings from above. Crawling was a painful operation. The coloring in these caves was red, brown, and black, with splashes of white.

I was glad to get out of that cramped cave. Camas wildly swished her tail, bobbed though it was, and jumped on me to show her enthusiasm for my escape.

In the evening, we headed out toward Broken Top. We hadn't walked all of Limbert's trail, but the weather had grown wild, with wind and a rare rain sweeping the land. Waist-high sagebrush made the way out harder--and wetter—than our entry had been, but we met a trail heading west at Trench Mortar Flat near the tree molds, those eerie rock models of incinerated trees that stood for centuries like banished ghouls. We were soaking wet and stopped to wait out the rainstorm in the shelter of Buffalo Cave. The remarkable rain kept falling in buckets in a parched landscape.

Not a person saw us arrive to the road in darkness. No one was the wiser about our illegal hike, nor about my sadness and joy in the wilderness. We were cold, wet, and miserable, but we had survived in style. We had seen the Craters of the Moon Wilderness, its virtues known by few. We climbed into my car, tired after two nights of camping and our marathon hike out. I was disappointed not to have made it to Laidlaw Park and decided to finish the rest of the hike in the summer.

***

In the summer heat of late July, Camas and I set out for Craters again, while Merritt was working. I wanted to know this monument in its least hospitable moments, which was not a feeling Merritt shared. I saw the landscape as lava-born, passionate, wicked, and alive, not a mere rock garden. This profound beauty Limbert had long ago conveyed to Congress. He too had found joy in the place called the bleakest on the continent.

Flowers, however, were on my mind as I drove from Boise through Carey to Craters of the Moon. I wanted to see how flowers in The Little Prairie compared with those in Laidlaw Park, the larger BLM kipuka to the south. Camas and I headed into the old monument hiking three miles through a'a lava, heading out of The Little Prairie and into the new monument and BLM land, climbing and crossing 5,900-foot North Laidlaw Butte on the way. The distance wasn't great, but the terrain was rugged and the temperature was rising from about 90 degrees Fahrenheit and would get extreme on black lava this afternoon. There were plenty of flowers nonetheless: buckwheat, antelope bitterbrush, dwarf monkeyflower, and larkspur, with their bluebird brilliance. Seeing the rich blue larkspur and the scarlet-pink monkeyflowers soothed me. They seemed defiant, like life, blooming in the middle of a raging fire.

Camas and I settled in for the night below Echo Crater. Behind the Pioneer Mountains, to our west, sunlight flamed orange under clouds and limber pines lined up along the horizon defining a flow of ancient lava. I woke up before dawn and looked south over The Little Prairie, wishing Merritt were here to see the beauty as I lingered in the morning glow. I planned to get an early start to beat the searing heat of afternoon, but as I rolled over to say good morning to Camas, she was nowhere in sight.

I called for her while I ate a peanut butter sandwich to assuage my hunger. I waited for Camas to come out of the somewhere she'd disappeared into, but she never did. I walked around in the stunted forest of limber pines and saw her tracks, along with others that I took for coyote tracks. There was no sign of a fight, but it was not like Camas to desert me. I laid my sleeping bag on a rise so I could see it from a distance and headed out to find her. I climbed up a small hill and called out her name, to no avail. Then I climbed Echo Crater to get a better vantage point.

Echo Crater provided a superb, if a bit confusing, view of Big Southern Butte to the east and North Laidlaw Butte to the south. From the crater's edge, a cauldron of rocky cliffs and limber pines dropped abruptly 500 feet into a cirque-like cup that was 400 by 600 feet in size. I walked the ridge of the crater calling, "Camas! Camas! Camas!" And I heard from below, "Camas! Camas! Camas!" Suddenly, I knew why it was called Echo Crater. Its beauty was unique and comical. I wanted to explore the floor of the crater, but the clouds were dissipating and my dog was still AWOL. I climbed back down and circled the camp, looking for signs of the worst, but I found none: no bloody carcass, no cougar tracks, nothing.

I waited for another hour, then two more. I kept calling Camas and searching for her. Finally, I decided to move on without her. Maybe I would find her along the route, but I felt heartless and I could almost hear what Merritt would say if I returned without Camas. The clouds were gone now, and I realized that the hot sun would be far more intense later when I was on the black lava hiking toward Laidlaw Park. I had to get going. I left Camas a bowl of water, built a rock monument as a memorial to her, walked on about a mile to the end of The Little Prairie, where I turned due south onto a thin peninsula of sagebrush. I bade farewell to my friend. She would never find me on this narrow route. It was an inglorious goodbye, as I dumped a gallon of the water that I'd been carrying for her. I now had about three quarters of a gallon to take me to the other side of the hot lava flow.

On the Dark Side of the Moon

Just as I made the turn into the narrow patch of sagebrush, Camas came running up out of nowhere, tired, happy, and thirsty. I was stunned. She must have smelled me and tracked me down to this point. I gladly gave her water, feeling like a murderer for leaving her behind. She greeted me with jumps and licks, and I welcomed her with a mixture of love, guilt, and relief at what I wouldn't have to live with. Merritt never had to know about this incident.

How selfish I had become! It was one more lesson for me to learn: not to leave my beautiful dog in this unforgiving desert. So we two pals traveled on. I thought I had enough water, but as The Little Prairie gave way to the a'a, the blistering sun and lava made me anxious. Did I really want to walk into the oven before us? An oven it was, heated from both the sun and the reflective black rock. I had read that the temperature just above the lava can reach above 140 degrees Fahrenheit, but I didn't carry a thermometer to give a number to my misery. Why, exactly, was I going here? Why would anyone go through the lava in the monstrous summertime heat? We moved slowly to the other side of the lava.

Camas and I crossed two miles of lava, shuffling up and down across sharp, jumbled pieces of jagged rock that clattered like wind chimes with every step. I couldn't imagine what barefooted Camas felt. We stopped at every tree that held a bit of shade, both to rest from the relentless sun and to avoid the blowtorch wind, but the trees were few and far between, often a quarter mile from one to the next. At a large limber pine, a great horned owl flew out of the sheltering canopy and off across the lava. The owl would have to fly a long way to find another shady perch and it flew until it was a speck on the sky. I thought of the owl in my vision in Boulder. It had promised to lead me to where I needed to go. Camas and I would stay here for a few hours in this small refuge, courtesy of the owl. It had given its spot for us here in the shade and vanished, here in the most unforgiving wilderness.

Camas heaved in the heat. She ran from one bit of shade to another across the field of lava, finding rabbitbrush, bitterbrush, and large, shading rocks to hide behind. I didn't want to torture her, and in the shade of the big limber pine we slept for an hour and a half, hoping the temperature would drop. It seemed to rise. As we lay there, I watched a pair of small birds flitting in the branches of the tree. I envied their energy in this blazing heat. I was sweating hard, but the sweat evaporated almost as quickly as it dampened my T-shirt. Camas panted heavily even in the shade. I got up to check the conditions for walking, and the sun slammed down on my shoulder like a flaming blanket. I eyed the amount of water that was left. A dog and a man drink much more than a man alone, and I had dumped most of the water because of the weight before Camas found me again. It might be enough. I ducked back into the shade, and we waited another hour before heading out into the cruel sunlight. With alarming sloppiness, Camas lapped a cup water that I'd set beside her.

As I lay down on the ground, my hazy consciousness turned to Limbert and my father. Both of them were roughly my age when they died, and here I was, stupidly hunkered down below a pine tree in the heat, thinking about what it might be like to die out here. Dehydration, blood flowing slowly and thickening into slushy globs, my heart struggling to push the blood to my brain and lungs, arms and legs going limp, body temperature rising, mind deluded by mirages and hallucinations, and then my heart or brain failing, a clot stuck in the flow, and life would stop. I knew better than to wait much longer. Even the worst cook knows to pull his loaf of bread out of the oven before it burns. I was burning. I blessed the water.

"Camas, let's get going," I muttered. "It's cooler now." That was a bit of wishful thinking. She wasn't fooled by my optimism. Darkness would overtake us in four hours, and I didn't want to camp in the harsh a'a lava field with so little water, especially since I partially blamed my stroke on a lack of water. It was still well over a hundred degrees and the black rock sent visible heat waves upward. In four hours, the air would be chilling. I craved water, popped a second aspirin in my mouth, and tried to remember if the moon would be full tonight. If so, I could walk at night; if not, I would have to sit tight and wait until tomorrow. I couldn't remember. Damn it; I couldn't remember! Camas moved reluctantly and drooped as we walked through late afternoon heat. I was convinced that there was never a worse time to walk in the lava, but walk we did.

I thought about Merritt in a feverish fantasy as we walked up and down through the brush and humps of lava. She was sweet and kind, funny and opinionated as a nanny goat. Nicely shaped, seductive, sexy, but with the linguistic venom of a sidewinder. Oh my, she could be cranky and direct, as I learned in our talks with a counselor. Hiring the counselor was a joint decision of ours, as we thought she would be able to help us diagnose and cure our problems. She encouraged me to speak about my feelings on having a stroke, and Merritt to talk of her fears and expectations of her future in this alien place. Neither bore fruit. She quickly told us to come back when we were ready to talk. "I can't do this for you," she said. "You've got to do some of the work for yourselves." We never went back.

Clearly I had decided to ignore the warning signals. I was excited about being married. But did I really want to be married? I wasn't sure, but the oppressive heat of Craters of the Moon in July, helped me grasp the present. I was only going to marry one woman, once in my life, and Merritt was the one who appeared in my greatest need. I wanted her to give me hope and to dance with me through this wounded life on our wounded planet. I wanted to forget the bullet holes in my mind and soul.

Age was no impediment for her. She was fearless in getting out of the morass of Washington, D.C., and coming to Boise, Idaho. She had a good job and was ambitious. I thought that we could pull off this life together if we shared our feelings and defined the roles we both could fill.

What could I give her? Surely it wasn't money, and it wasn't my clarity in thinking. She had been through an unexpected event herself, when her horse landed on her, and she lent me compassion. Was that enough to marry for? What did she want? Security? A child? A man around the house? I could provide those, yet I really didn't know what she wanted. And first I had to prove my worth to myself, because my self-worth had been decimated by the stroke. That's why I was out here in the desert. I would prove something to myself, to my father, and Limbert, both of whom, of course, were not there at all.

The lava was scorching with a brilliant obsidian shine. Everything growing out here had one purpose: survival. I had a journey—no path, but a journey--that I had to follow to find out why I existed after the stroke. I found no answer on the trip but heat and hardship. What I found was Camas, stark beauty, and myself in this blistering-hot desert, sweating and barely surviving once again. It was time to go home.

After another hour and a half of stumbling through piles of sharp lava, Camas and I made it to the kipuka of North Laidlaw Butte, pushing through thick, high brush to the grassy summit. The tall thickets gave us a reprieve from the sun, but it was work to get through. A pair of deer bounded off from under foot, and we discovered a tiny fawn lying motionless in the brush. Camas sniffed at it curiously. I pulled her away, and we continued walking. I was sorry to have scared the parents of this newborn fawn and hoped they would find their defenseless offspring. Of course they would.

Atop the butte another exquisite view spread out, this time of Laidlaw Park, an enormous tract of gray–green grassland surrounded by lava. Snowdrift Crater, visible as a slight line above the flat terrain, looked inviting at the north end of the big kipuka. That was our destination, but we had another mile of lava to traverse as the afternoon deepened into the slanting shadows of coming evening.

The mile took more time than I had anticipated and we traveled up and down more than straight. Our passage regularly dead-ended at punishing ridges of lava, forcing us to retrace our steps to a more promising route. I forgot any noble thoughts and focused on staying cool and saving what little water remained.

Exhausted but relieved, we arrived in the grassy north side of Laidlaw Park, where the hiking was easy and the grasses flowed like waves in the Pacific Ocean. Mercifully, the early evening cooled us on this long day and the moon was out and full, big and silvery as a lucky silver dollar. At the edge of the park, in Snowdrift Crater, a place seldom grazed by livestock or visited by people, a red-tailed hawk flew around and around the sunken, embracing cliffs. The land was dotted with tall grasses and chest-high sagebrush and many kinds of flowers: pentstemon, pussy-toes, white camas. We passed through a grove of aspen trees on the way through Snowdrift Crater, their leaves rattling in coolness. It wasn't exactly a biblical land of plenty, but I wondered how it had survived this ecologically intact. I thought about the old proposal for a well to be dug in the northerly Laidlaw Park area and realized why this land retained its value. There was still no well. I committed myself to holding out for the proposed Laidlaw Park Area of Critical Environmental Concern proposal in order to protect the vegetative community in the future. If the millions of acres north of the Snake River and south of Laidlaw Park ever again looked like this landscape, I would die a much happier man.

Just before dark, Camas and I were out of the furnace and back at the car. We drank as much sweet, sweet water as we could stand and I packed my gear into the car. On the way through Laidlaw Park, I stopped near an unnamed cindercone and marveled at North Laidlaw Butte, Echo Butte, The Sentinel, The Watchman, Fissure Butte, Sheep Tail Butte, Split Butte, and Two-Point Butte, all parts of a fascinating landscape now politically unified as the Craters of the Moon National Monument and Preserve. As we left the lava fields in Craters, the memories of Limbert and my father stayed, their ghosts had only come to guide me for awhile through the rugged terrain.

On a whim, I turned my car off and walked half a mile to look more closely at Big Blowout Butte, on the odd chance of spotting the falcon I thought might have been seen a year and a half before. I'd only had a glimpse of her right before I'd had my stroke, but there she was, or one just like her, flying in the crater of Big Blowout Butte! It was a prairie falcon; I was amazed to have found her, given the chances and the failing light. I can't say why I was so sure that she was a female, but I was. She was swooping and flying on quick wings, taking thin bites of air and calling "Ke-eek, keek, ke-eek!" She seemed to be telling me: "Go away! Go away! Go away!"

On the Dark Side of the Moon

I sat down to watch the bird. I was mesmerized by her quick, erratic, almost batlike, maneuvers, and I hoped her distress would abate. It didn't. She landed across the crater a quarter mile away and continued screaming at me. She was protecting something and didn't want me there, that much was clear. She must have had a nest somewhere in the lava cliffs, but I saw no mate and no young. I didn't want to continue bothering her and, in any case, the afternoon was quickly growing into night. I left the crater reluctantly, looking back at her and hoping she would live there for a long, long time. This landscape of disparate parts, from Inferno Cone in the north to Big Blowout Butte in the south, was one landscape in the eyes of the prairie falcon. She oversaw and guarded the land. It was her home and I understood her contentment.

**

We were back home now. Camas still climbed the tree out back in search of squirrels. My lack of a lucrative job and my money problems were our problems now, as all the little obligations came pouring back.   Life went on, and Merritt and I made the best of it. We argued about small things: the garden, planting trees, cutting the grass. And we compromised: the deck had to go, and the back bedroom needed new carpet but we couldn't afford it. The deck seemed enormous, but it was rotting into the soil, and tearing it up meant living in the dirt in barbeque season and trying to rebuild it when we could afford to do so. "All right, let's get rid of it," I agreed. The back bedroom rug was stained, and we replaced it with another and didn't go out for dinner for awhile. "Ok, no Thai dinners," Merritt conceded. We agreed we would move if the opportunity arose. Neither of us gave in on much of anything; we were married to stubbornness like Fred and Wilma Flintstone, but we were survivors.

An Unbearable Beauty

I was a beekeeper of roughly 100 hives, and Merritt and I worked together in the garden around our house. Tenacity, love for each other, passion, and love of the outdoors were the things we had in common. The opportunity to move to Salt Lake City for a better job arose for Merritt, and so we moved. We would use our profits from the house in Boise to pay for a mortgage in Salt Lake, and we could start a new life. Or at least that was the plan.

Before moving, I planned to head for Craters of the Moon with Camas as my confidant and witness for one last hike. I told Merritt this might be my last hike alone.

"Tell me where you're going." She didn't want to worry about me.

"We're going ov-a to hike acro-ss the south side of the monu-nu-ment through a part of the Wapi Flow, head-ead to Kings Bowl and a little cave." I especially wanted to see Lariat Cave, mostly for its name, and I showed it to her on a good map to make it clear where we'd be. It had become a sore point when I took off without her on a trip to Craters, but I assured her that I'd only go alone this one last time. Craters had become a refuge for me with its solitude and time to think. I had learned a few secrets of the terrain in my peregrinations there, and I did want to share them with Merritt, but that would have to wait for now.

"Be careful," she said.

Camas barked. She always barked when she knew something was about to happen. As always, she was ready for a trip out to anywhere--ready for life.

"And don't kill your dog," Merritt added, only half--joking. I had told her about the last trip.

"Right." We kissed as I sat in the car with the window rolled down. "See ya day after ta-morrow." The bees wouldn't need keeping for a few days while I was gone. We were leaving them anyway and there would be other struggles to live through. Camas rode shotgun and watched everything that passed.

The Arco-Minidoka road was hot and dusty, and after our three-hour drive to the Wapi Flow, we climbed out at the southern end of the Great Rift. The Wapi Flow was formed 2,200 years ago in a single burst of volcanic activity and is more than 110 square miles in area. It is separate from the Craters of the Moon lava field to the north, but is connected by the Great Rift. Camas and I found a clear, cool day as we hiked into Crystal Ice Cave and King's Bowl. While they each looked spectacular to me, even grand, both had been damaged by careless use in the past. A rutted parking lot remained beside the original entrance to the Crystal Ice Cave, and the cave opening was a large hole with bars cemented to keep tourists out. The site was disappointing. We drove on to the weird, blown-out Pillar Butte at the heart of the Wapi Flow, and ended the day at remarkable Lariat Cave, so named because it loops around underground like a cowboy's twirling rope.

I entered into the cave's intimate darkness, bumbling along with another poor flashlight—my trademark, it seemed--that blinked out when I bumped it. I crawled like an earthworm into a narrow place, stood, and felt scared that I had gone too far back to return safely. The route twisted and looped into the darkness, and soon I felt confused in this tight lava space as I squeezed through the land, walking forward like a zombie. After a long time, whether it was fifteen minutes or an hour I cannot effectively estimate--I was lost in the disorienting darkness--I saw a spot of light. Was this another outlet? I moved quickly forward toward the light, as if navigating by the North Star.

An Unbearable Beauty

Camas sat outside the cave in the dim light. At no point had I been aware of walking this path to return to this spot; I mean, the path seemed to go straight and yet it had to curve around in a circle. That seemed impossible. The same exit had apparently been my entrance; I must have come full circle, walking the lariat. After climbing out, I sat in late afternoon light, astounded by the circumstance and comforting Camas. I realized that in this cave I found a valuable lesson about moving forward into the darkness.

We drove north for as long as the light held and found an unmarked place on the roadside to camp out beside the Great Rift. It wasn't much but it gave me a view of stars and land. Craters had once been characterized as "black vomit," a place only distinctive for the desire of wagon travelers to move on and settle elsewhere, in a more productive world. They had been impatient, suffered in the heat, and they had all gone away. But this last leg of the journey was my own, shaped by memories of my father, on a path set by Limbert, and with the love of Merritt, my mother, and all of the women and men who have loved me, in their unique ways. I was thankful to each of them in my broken way.

The night was lovely, clear, and warm, with a slight breeze from the west. The full moon shined with a whiteness that filled the scared land with light and shadow. Then the earth eclipsed it perfectly, darkening slowly to near totality, and for hours the round moon glowed red. I saw the satellite moon in a new, remarkable way, and realized that the value of wild places is not what you can take from or add to them, but what you are given, free of charge, to learn from them.

Craters of the Moon is a place of fragile beauty and frank brutality, wonder and silence, dryness and wetness, savage heat and crystalline coldness, and it will call me back again and again.

On the Dark Side of the Moon

The landscape provided a mirror for my charred soul, and I now realize that it helped rehabilitate me far more than I ever helped Craters of the Moon recover. What I've learned, so far, is a profound respect for Craters of the Moon and myself, being just as they are. There is no God outside of me; it is within me, looking out with my eyes.

Molten rock running over the land 2,000 years ago has clotted and hardened to a crisp black covering and this land is still recovering into productive soil, but the process will be arduous, slow, inevitably partial. The topography reads hard, like a life. It is pocked with craters, hornitos, spatter cones, and fields of lava, but it is also full of surprises, like the soil-catching pockets and grasslands in the middle of acres and acres of rock. It is these places that give life.

An impatient part of me wanted to change the way the world worked in 15 minutes and make victories certain. It insisted upon naming defeat and success immediately. That part is now gone. To be sure, I am angry at outrageous fate and eager to protect more land from opportunism, but I realize that everything involves slow, evolutionary changes, whether in health or politics, wilderness protection, or love. Even concrete dissolves in time. Incremental changes are what we create, hoping that they are good enough for today, with the slim hope that today will last forever.

I feel wildness in the wind and imagine a curtain of fire erupting before me. Brilliant lava sprays up in powerful surges, yellow, red, and silver, a 500-foot vertical wall, 50 miles along a slim crack in the earth—the Great Rift. Smoke rises in billowing clouds as I watch the blinding brightness and smell the overwhelming bitterness of sulfur fumes. Loud explosions, like cannon blasts, jar my body as the fountain rises and falls and forces me to hide from the heat. Fire! A spontaneous, mesmerizing show dances, pulses, sparks, and glows, as unknowable as it is dangerous. Now it is still and burned--the smoking landscape in my head. When I open my eyes, I see nothing but a barren, glorious wilderness to explore and a moon drenched in blood.

Just as suddenly, the brightness returned. The eclipse of the moon has now passed as surely as my stroke has gone away, as surely as Lariat cave led me to continue moving forward into darkness. These are lessons of Craters of the Moon. I tell myself it has passed, but I will never forget the ox blood stain on the moon.

There is more time to think. It was not my desperate searching that led me to wellness and health, but my love of this land, all of my friends, my mother and father, Camas, Limbert, and Merritt who restored my broken spirit when I needed it most. And what would life be without the fire and ice, unknowable risk and unseen beauties, friendship and passion, the noise and silence, and the harsh sunshine of wild country? I can tell you, it would be utterly unbearable.

On the Dark Side of the Moon

AFTERWORD

As I drove beside Jughandle Mountain near McCall, Idaho by the Salmon River Mountains in 2012, I saw the green of a familiar meadow, with a brilliant burst of shooting star flowers in its midst. I pulled over to look at this ephemeral batch of colors and to bask in my luck at ever seeing them at all. Shooting stars look just like they should, with a brilliant yellow tip out front and purple petals streaming behind. It is a miracle to catch them in the blinking flight of summertime.

Merritt and I moved different ways as I continued to grow more confident in my recovery and she settled into her job as the executive director of the Utah Rivers Coalition. I took a job in La Grande, Oregon, out of a need to survive. She stayed in Salt Lake City, and we both grew tired of the long commute and my poor communication skills. We agreed to meet on a monthly basis, sometimes in Salt Lake City, and other times in Boise or La Grande. My job as executive director of Hells Canyon Preservation Council consumed me, as I struggled to communicate clearly with a diverse board of directors and the disenchanted staff of the organization. I had been hired by Ric Bailey, the mercurial and forceful founder of HCPC, and a board that mostly seemed confused. Ric was the soul of the organization, and he was headed out to live on a nearby piece of land in Enterprise, Oregon, the town where he had once been hanged in effigy. Enterprise had changed in ensuing years, mostly because of Ric's long-time presence beside this stunningly beautiful canyon with a rich history.

Merritt and I talked on the telephone at least every other night, and one night she suggested that we meet in Boise at a friend's place. It was a stylish condominium that overlooked the city and the dry foothills to the east. Neither of us was satisfied with our relationship, and we needed to discuss what we should do. I drove down I-84 to Boise from La Grande and she drove in from Salt Lake City.

She quickly got to the point: "Mike, I can't continue this relationship long-term. I want a divorce." Sublety was never Merritt's strong point.

"Oh, ok. I understand," I felt numb and broadsided.

"What do you think?"

I had never thought about a divorce, and I didn't want to bail out on my marriage. "I don't know." I diddled. "That seems pretty extreme. Is there anything that we could work out?"

"I guess. But we never see each other." I looked down. She continued. "You chose to live in a place without an airport nearby and it's a long drive. That's pretty limiting."

"Yeah. But the job is a gift that I couldn't pass up."

"*You* wanted to live in Salt Lake. We moved there together."

"And I couldn't make it there." I had a series of jobs that I could never seem to hold, and I saw the job in La Grande, Oregon as a familiar job in familiar territory.

"You didn't try," she said.

"I did."

Afterword

The only thing on which we agreed was that our relationship wasn't working, but neither wanted to really change to make it work. Both of us had ardent desires to succeed in our fields, and that afternoon, we both lost. I also lost my job in La Grande in six months, and moved back to McCall, Idaho, where I had lived 15 years before.

Many of my old friends live in this long valley in McCall. It's a gorgeous place, and I feel my great good fortune in being here. Twelve years ago, I had a devastating left-sided stroke, and now I finally feel that I am moving on. I finally find myself once again a writer, an environmentalist, and a man with strong opinions. It wasn't as big a change as I had once feared.

When I first had the stroke, I thought, *What a great reason to write about my experience of having a stroke in Craters of the Moon!* And it was. Fortunately, I've kept my journals on the experience. Unfortunately, it wasn't nearly as easy as I had hoped to write about this journey. It has taken me more than a decade to write this story, during which I forgot and lost much, but gained more. After the stroke separated my past life from the present, I had to ask myself, *Who am I? Whom have I become after 55 years?* I really didn't know who I was at all, which is a significant problem for a writer and professional environmentalist. Or anyone else, for that matter.

For me it has been a privilege to have had, survived, and then returned from a stroke. I saw childhood as an adult, saw worlds that I hadn't ever imagined, and found out what hard work really is. Today, I am lucky to be able to stand, speak, run, think, see, hear, move, and to love. It's a lot to be grateful for.

Wilderness has always been part of my life, and will continue to be. When I say "wilderness," I mean truly wild landscapes, big expanses which beckon me to travel further away from city life. As I mentioned earlier, Henry David Thoreau wrote, "In wildness is the preservation of the world." This is what being in the wildness of Craters of the Moon offered: the preservation of my world. Wilderness is the humble place where I can always learn, where I am always brought to peace regardless of the turmoil of my life. Go to the wilderness and you will find the ability to recover and heal yourself.

Family, friends, beauty, and nature were the reasons that I survived and prospered in the face of having a stroke and the outrageously slow recovery that has followed. At times death would have been easier, and this life of mine could simply end peacefully. However, Craters of the Moon cradled me for several years when I needed to feel the solitude and see the beauty in this dead-seeming landscape of lava. What I thought was dead wasn't dead at all. Craters and I both needed restoration and both posed an impossible task. It was, and is, a fight to be fully alive.

Recently, I read the brand new Record of Decision finalizing the Craters of the Moon National Monument and Preserve Management Plan. It was long in coming and when it came, it offered substantial improvement on the management that was in place before the establishment of the monument in 1924. The greatest change that the monument creation process brought was in one simple statement: "There will be no new livestock developments permitted in the North Laidlaw Pasture or Bowl Crater." According to this plan, Laidlaw Park would not be further degraded, and in time the ground and all its life, would recover. Perhaps not as it was, but in time, Craters will recover to a new self.

Afterword

On the Dark Side of the Moon

Acknowledgments

Thanks to Lynae Nielson, Doug Schnitzspahn, Katie Fite, Char Roth, Miguel Fredes, Ralph and Jacki Maughan, Christie Babalus, and Scott Groene for their love; to Mary "Chocolate-Moose" Jones (for rides, encouragement, and superb pastries in the middle of the night), John McCarthy, Pat Ford, Belinda Bowler, Dr. Steve Asher (for his remarkable insights), Amy Haak, Matt Mayfield, Kim Howard, Jim Cockey (for time, space, and thoughts), Dave McElwain who gave me remarkable acupuncture for my soul and body, and Debra Purcell, for her compassion in all of life.

For remarkable editing (and far too little pay) my appreciation goes to: Joy Johannssen, Katie Alvord, Kate Baxter, Joanne O'Hare, and Kelly Luce. And for all of my writing friends who endured despicable drafts and helped turn all of the gobblygook into a book with their thoughtful suggestions; they include Alvin Greenberg, Doug Schnitzspahn, Nick O'Connell, Tim Palmer, Steve Trimble, Rocky Barker, Rich Rahill, Mark Hengesbaugh, Clay Morgan, and Scott Gipson. Thank you to Brooke and Terry Williams, Cort Conley, and David Shields who gave me inspiration to move forward through darkness and to Governor Bruce Babbitt, Dr. Antonio Damasio, and Robert Limbert for providing a path toward the light.

As for the nurses, pilots, volunteer and professional EMTs who worked with LifeFlight in a nightime rescue from lava in Craters of the Moon: thank you; I owe you my life.

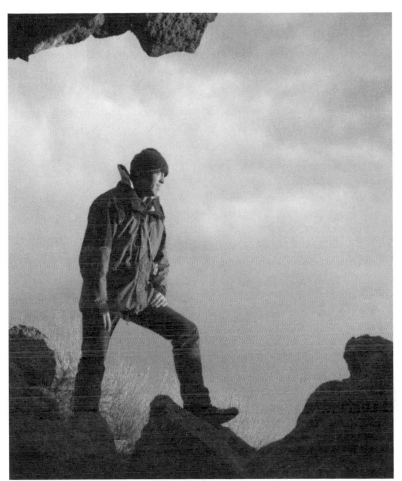

Mike Medberry has served as a senior environmentalist for several local and national conservation organizations, has an MFA from University of Washington, and has been published in many western publications over 25 years. He has written nonfiction for *Northern Lights Journal, High Country News, Black Canyon Quarterly, Hooked on the Outdoors, Wilderness Magazine,* and the e-magazine, *WritersWorkshopReview,* as well as short fiction for *Sun Valley Magazine, Boise Weekly,* and *Cold Drill.*

Thanks to Idaho Commission on the Arts for providing three crucial grants supporting graphics, and editing for my book.

Thank you to the following publications for printing my articles that are related to this book:

The Writers Workshop; *Craters of the Moon;* June 9, 2009; e-publication.
Stroke Connection Magazine; *A Stroke in the Craters of the Moon;* March/April, 2004 (cover story).
Sun Valley Guide; *"Craters of the Moon;"* Summer, 2003.
High Country News; *Ground Zero;* June 2003
Boise Weekly; *"Two Gun Bob"* and the *"Craters of the Moon;"* January 15-21, 2003.
Black Canyon Quarterly; *Stroke of Fortune;* Winter 2002.